CANDIDA AND ILL HEALTH

A DOCTOR'S EXPERIENCE

recounting a lifelong work on the
management of patients with
Candida Overgrowth

by
DR. RAY CHOY

text copyright © Ray Choy 2019

Published by Shimran
an imprint of Fitzrovia Press
www.fitzroviapress.co.uk

ISBN 978-0-9570722-7-5

printed and bound in Great Britain
by
Grosvenor Group Print Services Ltd
Essex IG10 3TS
text on FSC bookwove 80gsm
cover on 300gsm 2 Sided Board

DEDICATION

This book is dedicated to my lovely wife Nancy
whose continuous support is well appreciated.

ACKNOWLEDGEMENTS

My thanks to my sons Jason, Paul and David for their help in dealing with the technical aspects of the manuscript.

Special thanks to Mrs. Miriam Bartlett and Mrs Dawn Andrew for reading through the original draft and making suggestions to make the book more readable.

To my agent Susan Mears for getting this book into publication.

I also want to thank the various patients who wrote letters about their experiences and thus contributed to this book.

ABOUT THE AUTHOR

Dr. Ray Choy graduated in medicine in 1974 at the University of Singapore. After working in Singapore for 3 years, in hospital and general practice, he went to Australia. In 1977 after 1 year of practicing family medicine in Australia he came to the UK. After a further 4 years of working in different hospitals he joined a practice specialising in medical conditions due to various environmental factors then called clinical ecology.

In 1987 he started his own practice looking at chronic ill health due to environmental reasons. His patients include people coming from different parts of the world and of differing social standing. He has been invited to several countries to see high ranking officials of those countries for their medical problems.

In 2002 he was conferred the Datoship (Malaysia State Knighthood) by HRH the Sultan of Pahang, Malaysia, where he was born, in recognition of his approach to treating patients with chronic ill health.

CONTENTS

.

FOREWORD I

by a Hospital Consultant Physician

I am indeed honoured that Dr. Ray Choy has asked me to write the foreword to his book on Candidiasis.

Dr. Ray and I go a long way back to 1962: I have known him since age 12 and had gone through school and medical studies with him. He has always been straight and honest; and coming from a humble background, always been very focused.

After graduation from University, whilst I did more exams to becoming a consultant physician, he took a different path. He spent time on looking at chronic medical cases with a different slant so that a plausible solution can be found. After 35 years, he has condensed his work and recollected his experiences in this book. I can testify to the validity of his approach as I have used it over the years alongside the conventional methods to the benefit of a lot of my patients. He has not advocated an alternative method but rather one that can complement the standard orthodox approach to chronic medical cases.

My encounter with this approach started many years ago. My wife had a chronic cough and after much investigations was given a label as having cough due to stress. I did not concur with that diagnosis. Also at about that time, my son was diagnosed as having a skin condition due to allergy of unknown cause. It was then that I packed my bag to seek the answers from London. I got a clinical attachment in King's College Hospital in London, where I thought would be the best place to get solutions. The answers were not to be found there and as fate would have it the answers that I was looking for were with the person I was staying with; namely Dr. Choy.

He has pioneered a uniquely simple yet effective way of diagnosing and treating chronic ill-health problems. Abundant thoughts are given to the pathogenesis, various signs and symptoms of the conditions. Candida overgrowth plays a key role in lots of conditions. The conventional diagnostic tools of skin testing and blood tests measuring IgE and IgG levels do not confirm the diagnosis nor dismiss it. The cost of clinical trials is prohibitive and only the pharmaceutical companies can afford it. Even a much successful and heralded drug trial does not bear up in the longer run and has to be withdrawn. The various initial successful trials with the Statin group of drugs are examples of this. There are many doctors now who question the use of this drug.

Medicine has made leaps and bounds since we were medical students and will continue to do so. This is more so in the field of surgery where new techniques and equipments have advanced this area. In the field of internal medicine, even though there are newer blood tests and investigations as well as more knowledge about diseases and newer drugs used, the approach is still the same. When investigations have ruled out any life threatening condition, then the patient will have to put up with the chronic symptoms and drugs are prescribed to combat them.

Medicine is taught and practised on evidence-based

principles which are gathered and collated after several trials and studies by different doctors. It must be recognised that parameters used are for a large group of patients and may not be suitable or applicable to any single individual as each individual would have different environmental factors and different biochemical make-up. If over a number of years, a great number of patients respond positively to an approach, then there must be some correlation with that method even though the number of patients and doctors involved are not as large as in conventional trials. (there are now doctors in research who are looking at medical problems from a similar viewpoint). In time when more doctors adopt this approach and report their results, then this will become acceptable in conventional medicine.

I have sat with Dr. Choy in his clinic and was astounded by the number of patients who have benefitted from his approach and treatment. I then resolved to learn more about this. He was generous with the sharing of his experience and I eventually learned it. His parting advise was that we must not trumpet the success to our colleagues yet till we get much more anecdotal evidence as it may colour their opinion of us negatively. (The Candida problem is not in the standard medical textbook).

This book is a result of 35 years of seeing patients with the approach and he is now ready to share his beliefs. I have used that approach alongside conventional methods in cases where I am stuck and that had yielded good outcomes.

It is well known that our foods do contain synthetic nutrients such as those available in the shops. The chapter on food-state nutrients help to clarify a lot of misconceptions.

His method of treating allergies and treatment with high dilution neutralising drops and the use of the muscle testing technique to identify the offending agents have proved to be practical and successful.

The dictum of our Alma Mater is firstly not to do any harm to our patients and Dr. Choy has just done that with his understanding and treatment of chronic illnesses.

I believe that in time the medical world will acknowledge his grasp of Candidiasis in chronic illnesses.

Dato Dr. M. K. Wong DIMP, AM, MRCP
Consultant Physician, Makhota Hospital
Malacca, Malaysia.

FOREWORD II

by a Professor of Nutrition

Dr. Ray Choy is an exceptionally gifted pioneer. He is amongst the early doctors to develop the management of patients with ill health due to environmental factors and is now an accomplished medical practitioner specialising in holistic health. Dr. Choy works to get to the root cause of illnesses and not just treat symptoms. For over 35 years he has held the view that our good health is synergistic with the good functioning of our digestive system. Our gut function and digestive system is key to absorbing essential nutrients such as vitamins, minerals, amino acids and many other beneficial nutrients that contribute to good health. This book offers excellent advice regarding how we can look after our digestive system and how to treat a compromised digestive system. A common digestive system disorder experienced by an estimated 33% of the population is Candida overgrowth and proliferation. This condition often lies at the root of many common physical and emotional ailments.

This detailed book shows us how to help ourselves achieve a better digestive system and overall improved health. Dr. Choy offers readers a comprehensive guide to understanding the factors contributing to Candida overgrowth in our digestive system. He gives the readers very practical steps regarding dietary intake and dietary reforms to improve the digestive system and our good health.

This is a unique book by an inspiring and dedicated doctor. It will provide the reader with information that can help improve your own health and reduce the burden of Candida within your digestive system. There is no question that the advice and information Dr. Choy shares in this special book is easily accessible and practical and can lead to better health.

E. Llewellyn
Microcosm Professor of IntegrativeNutrition
Beijing University

PREFACE

HOW THIS BOOK CAME ABOUT

Why another book on Candida? There are already several books on this subject in the bookshop and some information is available on the internet. Yes, but what I have written is based on observations about actual patients, and what I have learnt from them and what they have told me about the Candida problem over the last 35 years. I have not stated anything new that is not known to others. This book is not based on any conducted trials or research but on clinical experience. It is not a rehash of available material. Therefore some of my opinions are very much my own, based on my experience with these patients, and may be at variance with what is generally said about this condition. I am not saying that the views and methods used by other practitioners are incorrect- they have their own preferred practises based on what they have been taught and the experiences they have gathered. So have I. And I am just putting that down in writing so that you may identify some of the varied symptoms that patients present with and start to understand this Candida problem.

The world was first alerted to Candida by Dr. C. Orian Truss in the late 1970s and then in his book called 'the missing diagnosis' published in 1982. He pointed out that doctors miss the diagnosis of chronic yeast infection which can account for a great deal of patients' chronic medical complaints. Since then various people have written books on Candida and subsequent authors repeated what others had stated before them but in a different style of writing.

In the early days of Candida treatment it was thought that environmental and food yeasts also contributed to the problem. Therefore, it made sense to avoid yeasty and mouldy foods and environment. In my experience this does not affect every patient. Hence it is not a routine avoidance. I have pointed out that only those who are affected by food yeast need to go on a diet of avoidance of yeasty or foods containing moulds as part of the make up. I have also highlighted a case in which environmental yeast played a big part in the symptoms. By and large it is not inevitable that there is a routine association.

This book is a reflection and recollection of the cases of patients with the Candida problem that I have seen over the years. I see patients with all kinds of medical complaints but the majority of them can be diagnosed as having a Candida problem. The Candida problem having been treated successfully resulted in resolution in their medical complaints, and as far as the patients are concerned, that is what they are interested in—to be free of their adverse symptoms. Most of them are not bothered with how the Candida overgrowth affected them or how the diagnosis was reached—as long as they get better with the treatment.

As this is not intended to be a medical text or a novel it is not written in a literary style, nor does it contain lots of medical jargon, but is very simple and understood easily. It is what I would say to my patients. This is not a big book about facts and research on Candida. It is just about my experience with the Candida problem: symptoms, treatment and response based on the patients I have seen over the last 35 years. Each case history or letter I have used in this book is to back up a point I have made, and took place in a true life situation.

Candida overgrowth is a very common problem and is a cause of chronic ill health especially where thorough investigations are negative for other conditions. It is also a factor in some diagnosed conditions which has not responded as well to treatment as expected.

Over the years I have seen quite a number of patients from different parts of the world and from different social circles, who also have a Candida problem. So the Candida problem is not just a western 'disease' or a condition of the more socially privileged, but is also seen in people from other parts of the world and in different social standings. My patients are people of all ages, professions and social standings, and it is clear that this condition is not prevalent in just one type of person from a particular environment.

The idea of writing this book was first put to me some years ago by a patient. She had remarked that my regime for treatment of her Candida problem was straightforward and easy to follow, and more importantly her problem was sorted out in a very short time. She had been on a strict diet which she found difficult to live with and had not got better from it with other practitioners. She suggested that I should write about my approach to the Candida problem. Over the years a few other patients have also made similar remarks. It wasn't till recently when I gave a short talk to some colleagues on the Candida problem that it was strongly suggested that I should put my views and treatment method in writing. So I am putting my experiences of this problem down on paper in the same way as I would discuss the Candida problem with my patients when they come to see me in my office. I am referring to the symptoms and consequences of the Candida overgrowth or imbalance as the Candida problem. The Candida species most commonly involved is Candida Albicans, though other species of the Candida genus can also be involved sometimes.

Most of my patients seek help because they have persistent unexplained ill health and adverse reactions to a large number of everyday substances. They have often suffered for years with what they assumed was incurable, such as irritable bowel syndrome, food intolerances and a feeling that they are 'allergic' to many things. Neither they nor their medical advisers had realised that in almost all cases, their symptoms are related to an undiagnosed overgrowth of the intestinal fungus – Candida Albicans. The imbalance caused by the overgrowth can be quickly and painlessly restored, and the previously persistent symptoms and ill health can be resolved within weeks. My patients then learn how to avoid or deal with future episodes of imbalances, and can live normal lives again.

Food forms a very important part of our life. We eat on average three times a day to keep us alive and functioning well. Eating and drinking also form a significant part of our social life. To give up your favourite food for a considerable length of time requires a great deal of discipline and in some people this can be very distressing and can be socially isolating. It is important to realise that, whilst the condition will respond somewhat to a very strict dietary regime, the rigidity in keeping to the diet may create another problem such as stress. And stress can make the problem worse. So on balance the patient does not gain positively by trying to stick to a very strict dietary regime, especially for longer periods. In my experience the best results come when practitioners treat the patient with the condition, and not just the condition itself. It is imperative to treat the person appropriately and not just prescribe the right regime for the Candida overgrowth.

One of the main reasons for writing this book is to raise awareness of just how prevalent undiagnosed Candida overgrowths are in this modern age, and to show how a Candida overgrowth can give rise to multiple symptoms, often resulting in ill health. In turn the treatment prescribed for the original illness often can exacerbate the original Candida problem, giving rise to long term unresolved ill health. If the Candida overgrowth can be diagnosed sooner, a simple and inexpensive course of treatment would see overall improvement in health and complete disappearance of the secondary symptoms due to Candida. I hope to be able to demystify and simplify for the public the understanding of the Candida overgrowth problem. Some patients believe, or have been told or have read, that a Candida problem can lead to very serious ill health and even to cancer. I do not believe this to be so. The underlying factors which promote the Candida overgrowth may contribute to serious ill health but the overgrowth itself is generally not responsible for other concomitant medical conditions, which need to be treated differently in order to ameliorate symptoms. It is important to bear in mind that there can be other concomitant medical problems with a Candida overgrowth and that one has to be aware of that, as other problems may need to be treated differently so that full resolution of symptoms be achieved.

I have reproduced several letters from grateful patients to highlight a few symptoms which can be related to the Candida problem. They have given their permission to have their letters printed in full though of course the names have been changed to protect their identity. Those whose names have been abbreviated have also had their initials changed. They are nevertheless real people with real stories and their case histories are used to emphasise the points made.

At the end of this book is some information on foods to avoid when on specific diets. This is not a book on recipes and therefore none are provided, except with one example in relation to a yeast free diet. I do not want to over emphasise the role of diet in this condition. Though it has a strong supporting role in the treatment of the Candida overgrowth, I do not consider it so very important in the treatment that you have to adhere to a diet strictly, but it is a relevant prong in the management.

This is not a book about the 'good' foods you should eat for good health but on dealing with the Candida problem.

This book is not intended to be a book on self-diagnosis or treatment. Any severe or persistent symptom must be investigated and you should see your doctor. It is only when acute medical conditions and serious illnesses are excluded and investigations are negative that one should then consider the possibility of the Candida problem being the basis of the symptoms. Tests can rule out what conditions you have not got, but the doctors may not be able to tell you what your underlying problem is and how to get you better. The Candida problem is not in the standard medical textbooks and so medical students who then become doctors are not 'raised' on awareness of the Candida problem.

It would appear that I have repeated a few things in different sections of this book. It is deliberate as I want to place emphasis on them. It is also very important for the readers to be reminded of those things and the reasons for me saying them.

Disclaimer
This book reveals the author's experience in dealing with the Candida problem over 35 years. The views expressed are his alone, gathered over a number of years seeing patients with the Candida problem, and can be controversial to other practitioners and especially to doctors in mainstream medicine. It is not a book on self diagnosis.

This book is not intended to replace medical advice. Any prolonged symptom that you have must be ruled out for more serious underlying medical condition by your doctor.

The author is just relating his experience and highlighting the varied presentations of the Candida problem.

HISTORICAL PERSPECTIVES I

PROGRESSION OF IDEAS

I first began to see patients with chronic ill health problems 35 years ago. Then I was working at a clinic which looked at conditions related to environmental factors as the cause of their symptoms. In using the phrase the 'external environment' I am referring to conditions such as hay fever, dust mite allergy, or exposure to common household chemicals like formaldehyde. I am not referring to industrial pollution. The internal environment relates to the food and drink we put into our body. The state of the micro-organisms in the intestine is very important to our good health, and the Candida balance with the other bacteria is of particular significance—though not too much emphasis was placed on that then.

Maimonides, a twelfth century physician, was attributed with the saying that 'one man's meat is another man's poison.' This means that food which is suitable for one person may cause adverse and inappropriate reactions in another person. I endorse Mamonides's view. This does not include some foods which contain toxic substances that may cause symptoms to most people. I am also not talking about a condition such as food poisoning due to bacteria toxins. It is the everyday foods which are tolerated by many but not by some people.

This view can be extended to include external environmental agents in our present day and age. What this means is that some people cannot cope with the things that others can, such as perfumes and air fresheners or pollens or house dust.

At that time I was seeing patients with reactions to a very wide range of allergens. These were usually patients who had seen many different specialists in different fields to try to find an answer to their medical complaints but to no avail. A whole range of tests had often been conducted but the results were usually unhelpful in determining what was wrong with them, and therefore the general conclusion reached by doctors was that the patient was suffering from stress, 'nerves' or depression. These patients usually ended up seeing a psychiatrist and being given antidepressants to combat the symptoms. These patients with chronic ill health and physical symptoms for which doctors could find no cause could end up feeling depressed because no cause of their complaints was identified—this led to some patients being accused of exaggerating or even manufacturing their symptoms. Antidepressants did make them feel better for a while but they still had their physical symptoms. Those patients seemed to be intolerant to all kinds of things, both internal and external agents. The Americans would call them universal reactors or multiple sensitivities, and the press would label them as suffering from the 20th Century Syndrome because everything in the environment would seem to give them symptoms.

Testing for various allergens was by intradermal (skin) injections following a method modified by Dr. Joseph Miller in America called the provocation-neutralisation technique.

The patient is usually tested for a number of suspected allergens causing their medical symptoms and if certain allergens are deemed to give a positive reaction by the way the skin reacts to the injected allergen then a neutralising dose is given. This is determined by the injection of serial dilutions of the allergen until the right dose is reached. This is called the neutralisation dose. Treatment is by a subcutaneous (under the skin) injection of 0.05ml of the neutralisation dose of that allergen. In this way it is not uncommon for patients to test positive to twenty or more allergens. I have even seen patients who were 'allergic' to a hundred common things. The aim is that the neutralising dose which contains the treatment to the offending factors will help the patient cope better with the allergens when exposed to it. This method does help the patients feel better to a variable extent, but a lot of them still have the underlying complaints and need their treatment (injections) adjusted (titrated) regularly otherwise the symptoms recur.

At this point it is relevant to know the story of how food allergy came to the attention of the medical world. In 1948 Herbert Rinkel was a medical student in Kansas, USA. He suffered from rhinitis (runny nose), and various treatments that he had did not help the condition. He came from a farming background and his family would send him eggs regularly to supplement his diet. One day the eggs did not come and so he went without eggs for some time. He noticed that his rhinitis stopped after a few days. When the eggs eventually arrived he ate them as usual and after a few more days his rhinitis returned. He then started wondering if his rhinitis had any correlation with the eggs that he had been eating regularly in large amounts. So he stopped eating eggs and after a few days his nose cleared and when he ate eggs again the condition returned. Thus the correlation between foods and symptoms was made.

Over the years more doctors became aware of this correlation and various tests were devised to help diagnose and treat this problem, all of which have fallen into disuse now, such as the Coco pulse test and the Basophils Degranulation Test. They have been replaced with blood tests which are more accurate but nevertheless do not give a total correlation with the food/foods causing the symptoms. It must be remembered that things that test positive are not necessarily the cause of the symptoms.

The most reliable way to test is by food elimination, and then to challenge with the food subsequently. If you avoid the food that you suspect is causing you symptoms and symptoms abate, and then when challenged with the food the symptoms recur, there is then a strong correlation with that food and your symptoms. Doctors gradually included external environmental agents such as common household chemicals, pollens and fungi into this category. The next problem was how to treat these patients with such problems.

In 1963 Dr. Carlton Lee in the USA, who suffered from migraine, found that when he injected himself with a certain dilution of beef extract, he got a migraine attack straightaway. He then experimented with various dilutions and found that with certain other dilutions of the same beef extract his migraine lifted. Thus was born the provocation-neutralisation technique of testing and treatment. After several years of research, Dr. Joseph Miller improved and standardised this technique, now commonly called the Miller technique and used by many doctors to treat patients with allergy problems.

When patients follow this treatment of injections, they do feel better but they need their injections regularly to keep their symptoms at bay.

I thought then that there must be some underlying factor that we had missed and if we sort that out the patients would derive much more benefit from the treatment, and in time be able to come off the injections.

At this time in my career (1987) I decided to practice on my own. I was then able to focus more intensely on finding that underlying factor. After a while I began to realise that the relevant underlying factor was the status of the Candida in the gut. If that was in a state of imbalance or overgrowth it could cause a lot of medical problems, and in some patients the symptoms became exacerbated as well as other existing conditions becoming worse. Over the years I have learnt from my patients that if the regime of treatment is simple (especially the dietary restriction) they will follow it well and get a good response. If the diet is too limiting, they will abandon it after a while, because for some who lead a very active social life it becomes almost impossible to adhere to it constantly—therefore their response is not as good as expected.

I

INTRODUCTION

WHAT IS THE CANDIDA PROBLEM?

When I say to patients that their symptoms are due to a Candida overgrowth, of those who have heard of the term, a few have said to me ' Isn't that a fashionable diagnosis '. Whilst that term may be in regular usage it does not negate the fact that they have symptoms due to the Candida overgrowth syndrome. That this term is used by a lot of practitioners, is evident from the number of patients I have seen coming to me with that diagnosis, from other practitioners. They had been treated for that problem albeit unsuccessfully. That is why they have come to me hoping that I would sort out their problem.

Candida Albicans and other species commonly called 'yeast' belong to the larger family of Fungi. They are classed in botany under the Plant Kingdom though they do not manufacture chlorophyll and do not have leaves. They also do not have roots to receive water and nutrients but instead have enzymes to digest organic matters from dead plants and other 'dead' matters.They are just like other organisms in our body and they are found in everybody though I doubt they are part of our original make-up. We 'acquire' them at some point before we are born or at birth. Our immune system which normally ejects foreign 'agents' from our body has somehow learned to 'tolerate' them and allows them to stay in our body. They live mainly in the gastrointestinal tract and in the female they are also present in the vagina. They are also present in the other orifices in our body and on the skin. Normally that existence is peaceful and in harmony with the other friendly bacteria in the gut and the immune system, which also deal with any untoward effects and keep things under control. Due to a variety of triggering factors this balance can be upset and then the subsequent overgrowth of the Candida can cause us much distress. It doesn't matter what the original cause was. It is like a damaged roof in our house—whether the damage was initially due to fire, tornado, bomb or other reasons, it is uncomfortable to live in such a house. The factors that cause the damage could have been long gone, but you are left with a house with a damaged roof. The roof has to be repaired for you to be able to live in it comfortably. The same applies to the Candida overgrowth if that is causing ill health. It has to be sorted out in order for us to regain good health even though the original triggering factor has long since gone and been forgotten.

Doctors have struggled over the years to find a term that would describe the Candida problem in the gut. Terms like gut fermentation, and gut dysbiosis are being used but there isn't a term that has been agreed on by doctors who deal with this condition. Besides, other organs can also be affected. This is not just a gut problem with confined symptoms in the gut.

The physical manifestation of Candida had been noted

for a long time. As far back as the year 400 BC, Hippocrates mentioned a condition in the mouth, that is now known as oropharnygeal thrush. Since then and over the years various scientists have described similar conditions. Initially the fungus involved was assigned to the Monilia family of fungi. Even now, especially in the older medical textbooks, vagina thrush is still known in some writing as Moniliasis. It was not until 1954 that the causative agent was confirmed and classified as Candida and that name has been in use ever since.

Candida is normally present in our body as a unicellular yeast form and is harmless to us. When the factors for overgrowth are present,the Candida organisms change into the mycelia form which are multicellular and they develop hyphae (feet) which can invade the gut mucosa.This can be the systemic invasion with septicaemia and usually in those patients with a very compromised immune system such as patients with cancer, HIV/AIDS, or those on very powerful immunosuppressants. This type of systemic Candidiasis can be fatal - but this is not what this book is about. I am talking about the much less dangerous form of Candida overgrowth which causes us chronic ill health with many varied symptoms.

Normally there is a good balance between this form of unicellular Candida and the 'friendly' bacteria in the gut. It is reckoned that there are at least 100,000,000,000,000 microorganisms in the gut. It is thought that there are more than 350 different species of bacteria and collectively they can come up to about 3-4 pounds or more in weight.There are about 200 different species of Candida, but the one that this book is concerned with is Candida Albicans. Albicans refers to the white colonies that are seen when this specie of Candida is cultured in the laboratory using the agar medium.

There are about fifty known strains in relation to the human being but they do not usually cause problems. Other strains such as C.Tropical, C.Lusitaniae, C.Glabrata, C.Parasilosis and C.Krusei are of less relevance to our health, though they can be present in substantial amounts in people with a very compromised immune system, and they contribute to making the underlying condition worse. Thus, sorting the Candida problem out in these people would certainly help in the management of the underlying condition. There is a very strong association between the autism spectrum of illness and Candida Parapsilosis, and one of the pillars of treatment in this condition is the elimination of this Candida.

Besides the 'friendly' bacteria such as the Lactobaccillus and the Bifidobacter species keeping the Candida Albicans in check, the immune system also has a very important role in maintaining the Candida balance, so that even though Candida is present in the body it should not cause trouble. The immune control is thought to be regulated by an immune-suppressor gene for the Candida, and if the regulation is weak then it does not take much to upset the balance. That may be why patients from the same family can experience Candida imbalances much more readily than others. It is not thought that parents can pass the Candida problem to the children (in other words it is not infectious) but the gene involved in the control can be inherited. It is not a true genetic link in the sense that you are not bound to have the problem even if one of your parents suffer from it, if the triggering factors are not present—but you may be prone to developing symptoms from the Candida more so than other people. In those with a very strong suppressor gene it will take quite a few factors to trigger symptoms. Hence the triggering factors and the genetically linked suppressor control are very important. If the gene is strong people can go through life without any symptoms attributable to Candida, or maybe with very mild symptoms every now and then which do not warrant any medical attention.

It is thought that we 'acquire' Candida at birth through the passage down the birth canal. Candida then multiplies rapidly in the gut so that by 6 months of life most babies test positive to Candida on skin testing. The gut refers to the gastrointestinal tract from the mouth through the stomach, small intestine, large intestine and rectum to the anus. Though it is reasonable to believe that we acquire Candida through vaginal delivery, it does not explain Candida in those born by Caesarian section. I think the Candida antigens (and there are seventy antigens already recognised) must in some way pass through the placenta barrier from the mother to the baby during gestation. Whether that is correct or not we do not know yet, but this fact is not relevant to the treatment. What is important is that the overgrowth needs to be sorted out and when it is sorted out the symptoms related to it are ameliorated.

Not uncommonly many patients think that a Candida overgrowth is synonymous with yeast sensitivity. This is not so in my experience. Going back to more than 40 years ago, not much was known about the Candida problem. Candida Albicans and other species of Candida belong to the Yeast family just like the organisms in Baker's Yeast, Brewer's Yeast and other forms of food yeasts. At that time it was reasonable to avoid all forms of yeast in the treatment of the Candida problem. My experience on dealing with patients with the problem over the last 35 years had led me to believe that it not necessary to avoid all forms of yeast in most patients, except in those who are also sensitive to yeast. An analogy would be that we all belong to the human race, but men, women and children are not the same. We eat food yeasts but we do not eat Candida. Yes, it is true that some patients with the Candida problem can also have yeast sensitivity, just like others can have milk and wheat or other food sensitivity, but the Candida problem is just about Candida and not other types of food or yeast intolerance. This book is about how Candida toxins can affect you when the Candida Albicans changes from the harmless unicellular form into the more sinister form of multicellular hyphae. This is not a book about food allergy.

Most doctors believe that with the Candida problem there is presumed yeast sensitivity. Whilst that may be so, I have treated patients successfully by simply sorting out the Candida overgrowth and I do not worry too much about any yeast sensitivity or food yeasts, as these problems are secondary. If a patient has them as well, they will automatically be sorted out in most cases once the Candida problem is resolved. Only the patients know with certainty what foods give them symptoms when eaten. Whilst their observations are correct (only they know exactly what happened) the interpretation of their observations may not be what they thought. When the Candida overgrowth problem is there all kinds of foods can seem to affect them. It is like, if you have a wound on your body, anything that falls into that wound can hurt you. You can take steps to prevent those things from falling into the wound so that you do not get hurt, but the wound is still there. So the wound has got to be healed, then those same things do not give symptoms unless in the analogy they represent very sharp things.

2

TRIGGERING FACTORS

VARIOUS EVENTS STARTING OFF THE PROBLEM

There are many reasons why the symptoms are precipitated. Patients may have a mild or the odd symptom prior to their current complaint, but it was not bad enough to warrant their close attention and so it was ignored until the symptoms became severe. Whilst it is interesting to know what triggered the symptoms, it is not always easy to find it in the medical history. The fact that we do not find the triggers does not mean that they are not there. It just means we cannot find them. Some factors may have arisen a while ago and the resulting symptoms were mild and so the trigger may have been forgotten. The important thing is that this does not alter the diagnosis or the treatment.

a) Antibiotics

This is by far the most common factor for giving rise to a Candida overgrowth. Some patients may get the symptoms after just one course and others after repeated courses of antibiotics. It is well recognised in conventional medicine that women can get vaginal thrush after antibiotics but it is not so readily acknowledged that intestinal Candida overgrowth symptoms may often follow. It is highly likely that the antibiotics which are designed to kill the bad bacteria which are harming you can also kill the good bacteria in the intestine, which are beneficial in maintaining the balance of the various microorganisms in the intestine. Many people may have had antibiotics on repeated courses to combat infections in childhood. That may have caused a mild imbalance of Candida leading to very mild symptoms; but not alarming and therefore forgotten.

b) Stress

Though emotional and mental stress are more common as triggering factors, one must not forget physical stress such as working prolonged hours or flying frequently for work, partying or not resting adequately. There is also physiological stress such as that which occurs when combating straightforward problems like viral or other infections.

It has not to be forgotten that in some people the body functions very well at times of stress. But when the stress has subsided their symptoms then come on. Thus they do not see the correlation.

GM, 45 year old lady

Was a sub-manager in a financial investment city firm who was at odds with her company over working conditions. That started nine months prior to me seeing her. Five months into her stressful period she developed a severe allergic reaction, collapsed and was admitted to hospital. No cause for her symptoms was discovered and she was discharged. Very soon after that she also develop symptoms after eating various foods. These included itchy hands and feet, abdominal discomfort and bowel upset. The Candida overgrowth was treated and she was much better—but she only felt back to how she was when the verdict of the employment tribunal ruled in her favour.

c) Steroid cream
AJ, 14 year old boy

Had Eczema since infancy and has been using steroid cream regularly for more than 10 years. Last six months he began to complain of tummy aches and sluggish bowels. When the Candida overgrowth was treated the abdominal symptoms resolved and skin problem got much better and he was able to stop using steroid cream after a period of time.

Steroid tablets, which are often used to manage acute asthmatic attacks or skin problem or other conditions termed 'auto immune', are also common triggering factors in my experience. Whilst the drug is still needed, when the Candida overgrowth is controlled and the contributing symptoms as a result of the overgrowth subsides, then overall treatment can be reassessed.

d) Tummy upset
WK, 47 year old lady

Was well until an episode of tummy upset five years ago. That resulted in diarrhoea up to 5 times a day ever since. She also had headaches, tiredness, and abdominal discomfort. When her Candida was sorted out her symptoms abated.

BV, 34 year old lady

Had salmonella from food poisoning. Shortly after treatment for it, she developed other tummy symptoms. Investigations for her other tummy symptoms were all negative. The symptom disappeared when her Candida problem was sorted out.

Gastrointestinal upset due to tummy infections can cause imbalance of the microorganisms in the gut. The original cause may have been treated but the persistence of the symptoms can then be due to a Candida overgrowth because the antibiotics which were used to treat the original gut infection upset the Candida balance even further in the gut and resulted in Candida symptoms as mentioned above.

e) Food poisoning
DLS, 41 year old lady

Contracted mild food poisoning. The next day following the food poisoning developed mild swelling of her lips and face which got more frequent and severe over the next few weeks. She also had migraine which she saw her doctor for and was given the appropriate medications. Though the migraine was relieved the other symptoms of swellings did not go away. They only resolved when the Candida was treated.

f) Drugs - Roaccutane
CL, aged 26

Developed Candida overgrowth symptoms shortly after taking Roaccutaine for acne on the face. Roaccutane is a very powerful drug and is prescribed only when antibiotics which are routinely used in the treatment of acne by GPs fail to yield results. I am sure other powerful drugs can also trigger symptoms of Candida overgrowth.

g) Child birth and hormonal changes
PT, aged 46

This patient was well until after the birth of her second child 10 years ago. She then developed gut symptoms and was diagnosed as having irritable bowel. Endoscopy was normal except for a small polyp in the intestine which was not responsible for her complaint and she was treated symptomatically. When the Candida was treated her symptoms resolved.

It is also commonly seen that some young ladies on the contraceptive pill develop symptoms of the Candida problem. Older ladies of the perimenopausal age can also develop such symptoms. It is clear that hormonal fluctuations are a recognised triggering factor.

Uncommon triggering factors

h) Prednisolone and antibiotics ointment for eye problems
ANL, aged 33
She was well until she had the treatment for an eye infection. Vaginal thrush and tummy symptoms followed shortly afterwards. When treated for the overgrowth, symptoms abated.

i) Post inoculation
I have seen a few patients over the years whose Candida symptoms followed a course of inoculation for their travels abroad. This is not a common triggering factor.

j) Growth spurt in children
This does not apply to adults and only in children. It is not triggered by gradual growth in these children but by the sudden shooting up e.g. 2 or 3 inches in height over a short period of time, or when they attain puberty. They can develop symptoms including the Candida problem which they never had before. I am sure the various hormones

involved in that process do play a big part in the precipitation of symptoms.

The above factors were not listed in any particular order of importance or frequency of occurrence except those involving antibiotics. Some factors were mentioned to highlight how seemingly unimportant illness or events can trigger a Candida overgrowth.

The case of SA is interesting because even though a few triggering factors had been present for a long time, there were no symptom until the last factor was encountered. She had asthma from a young age and needed antibiotics for the chest infections which she had from time to time. At age 17 she had a parasite infection of the gut and was treated with antibiotics. At age 20 she started taking oral contraceptive, but she still had no bad Candida symptoms until the age of 24, when she encountered a lot of stress at work. This led to persistent abdominal gas and bloating and erratic bowel movements. The Candida problem was treated and symptoms subsided and she was able to return to work without recurrence of symptoms even though conditions at work remained as they were before. She subsequently left for another job and has stayed well since.

An interesting but very unusual triggering factor is that of MW. He was swimming in the sea and was stung by jellyfish. He was treated appropriately, but a few days later he found that wheat and many other foods upset him and caused breathing problems. When the Candida was sorted out he found that foods which used to upset him he can now tolerate without any adverse effects.

Women are more commonly affected by the Candida problem than men. The difference is the presence of the female hormones in women (oestrogen and progesterone), the hormone in the 'Pill', the fluctuating hormonal levels in the menstrual cycle and the increased levels of hormones during pregnancy - all these are triggering factors.

One factor that is uncommon but has been cited by some researchers is the mercury from dental amalgam fillings. This is especially so in those patients whose Candida problem does not respond to the usual treatment or who have frequent recurrences. It seems that the mercury vapour from the amalgam reacts with the hydrochloric acid in the stomach to form mercury chloride which is toxic to bacteria. As a result the function of the 'good' bacteria in the gut is undermined and this allows the Candida to proliferate.

I am sure there are some other less common and unusual triggering factors. It is not important to know the exact cause if you cannot find it, but important to get the correct treatment for the problem.

3

SYMPTOMS

DIFFERENT CLINICAL MANIFESTATIONS OF THE PROBLEM

Candida fermentation produces toxins. These toxins can affect any system in the body. Patients often have multiple symptoms and those who present with a single complaint often (when asked the right question) reveal lots of other symptoms. They are aware of these symptoms but do not mention them either because they are not aware of that the various symptoms are linked or because they do not view them as being as important as their main presenting symptom.

1) Digestive tract disturbance – the most frequent symptom

i) Tummy bloating, gas, or feeling windy, burping or flatulence, dull tummy ache or acute colicky pain—these are the most common complaints. Sometimes when they have these symptoms for a long time, they learned to put up with them as they are not life threatening and do not mention them as those symptoms have always been there for a long time and has become part of them. What I have heard very commonly is that when they wake up in the morning the tummy is flat. But as the day goes on the tummy becomes more distended so that by evening they look pregnant. In fact with some younger ladies they have been asked about the pregnancy.

When you are sleep you do not eat for 6-8 hours and so the tummy is flat in the mornings. As the day progresses we put in cumulatively more foods into our tummy. Almost everything we eat breaks down into sugars in our bodies, so more and more fermentation occurs with the resulting tummy distention.

ii) *Bowel disturbance—constipation or frequency of bowel movements with diarrhoea, erratic bowel movements with alternating constipation and diarrhea, hard or watery stools.* There should not be any blood in it unless there is concomitant haemorrhoids or anal fissures. If blood is tinged with the stool without any obvious reason than further investigation will be needed to exclude more serious conditions such as colitis.

iii) *Acid reflux or heartburn*—patients are often on anti-acid medication given by their doctors for this symptom. I have seen enough patients with both this symptom and a Candida overgrowth to make me wonder what links these conditions and after lengthy observation I noticed that the 'acid' problem disappeared when they had recovered from their Candida problem—unless they had an underlying hiatus hernia. My own theory is that the gas resulting from the fermentation travels towards the stomach and distends it. This stretches the cardio-oesophageal valve: this valve is found at the lower end of the oesophagus and the stomach, and prevents the stomach contents from going upwards back to the oesophagus normally. Thus the hydrochloric acid produced by the stomach stays in the stomach and does not travel up the oesophagus where it can damage the lining with prolonged exposure. The cardio-oesophageal valve gets stretched and does not close so competently due to a bloated stomach. The gas gives the stomach a greater pressure than the oesophagus, which forces the stomach acid to go upwards. When the Candida problems are sorted out there is minimal gas production and the stomach is not distended, and therefore the acid does not travel upwards to the oesophagus. The cardio-oesophageal valve stays closed properly and does the job that it is designed to do, and so the acid reflux symptoms subside. Whether this is the right explanation or not I do not know but it is certainly a plausible explanation for the improvement in those patients.

Nausea or vomiting happen because of the increased pressure in relation to outside the body. The only way to equalise the pressure is to open up the cardio-oesophageal valve and throw up.

IBS or Irritable Bowel Syndrome is a very commonly used term for those with tummy or bowel complaints where various investigations have turned out negative. It is important to know what you haven't got like cancer or intestinal obstruction, though they (the doctors) may not know what can account for your complaints. These symptoms are usually made worse or precipitated by various emotions such as feeling stressed, sad, or even excited. They that diagnosis in accordance with what they have been instructed in lessons on gastroenterology, even when told (by the patient) that eating makes their symptoms come on and the tummy feels much better when the patients haven't eaten. When the Candida is treated these symptoms usually subside.

2) Skin problems

i) Eczema—very common. Orthodox doctors do not see the link with what patients are eating and the condition of their skin. Treatment using steroid creams of varying concentration can suppress the skin condition but the underlying cause is still there, so the patients have to use the cream for a long time with resultant side effects. Now, with the advent of a non steroid based cream, more doctors are using it with various degrees of success. But what about treating the underlying cause?

ii) Acne in adults. Those patients have usually been on drug treatment such as Antibiotics and Roaccutaine to treat the problem. The skin can look good when they were on those drugs, but when the course was finished or was stopped then the acne reappeared after a while. Whilst it is not a life threatening condition but to the young adults especially girls, it is unattractive and can cause depression.

iii) Urticaria (wheals) with or without accompanying angioeodema (puffiness of skin tissues generally). This is also a very frequent condition that I see and they respond very well with sorting out the Candida problem. In fact some patients have this problem for a long time and their doctors told them that they have chronic urticaria and will need medication for a long time. I can state that to date, I have not fail to treat successfully urticaria in my patients.

iv) Skin rashes and itchiness without a skin rash. It is important to exclude the more serious underlying pathology such as cancer.

v) psoariasis—this is not an uncommon problem that I see from time to time. Though other factors can also trigger off or exacerbate existing psoriasis such as stress and absence of sunlight, sorting out the Candida problem when present will lead to amelioration of the skin problem to a varying degree. How much better the skin will get will depend on how much the Candida contributes to the underlying cause. These patients will get better and together with the management of other factors I have had cases of full recovery. It is just that we cannot predict the extent of the recovery. Creams and other medication and Vitamin D do help to resolve the acute skin condition for that moment, but dealing with the underlying factors can lead to more permanent relief.

3) Lethargy and tiredness

Though there may be other reasons for this, Candida toxins can account for those complaints. One of the products of fermentation is alcohol: like the patients drinking small amounts of alcohol throughout the day. In fact a very common observation is that patients complain of a 'hangover' when they wake up in the morning even though they have not been drinking any alcohol. These are very common symptoms presenting alone or in conjunction with other symptoms. Of course anaemia and a low functioning thyroid and others can also cause these complaints and these need to be ruled out. Mineral deficiencies can also contribute to these symptoms.

4) Decreased mental clarity and concentration

The most common phrases patients used to describe these symptoms are 'spaced out' and 'brain fog'. They also said that they could not concentrate well or their brain was not working as well as it should.

5) Mood swings

Fluctuating moods and emotions with periods of feeling 'high' and periods of feeling 'low'. Could this be related to the wildly fluctuating blood sugar?

6) Intense cravings for carbohydrate and sugar

These two symptoms I feel are linked very closely. They result from wild fluctuations of the blood sugar levels, I think. Normally our blood sugar fluctuates smoothly. When we have eaten our blood sugar goes up. When we are hungry this is a sign that the blood sugar is coming down, so we eat to bring the blood sugar up again. Our body releases sugar or converts stored glycogen into sugar to maintain the blood sugar level so that we continue to function well even when we cannot eat for some time. In some people and in those with the Candida problem, this mechanism does not seem to operate or work so well,and so the blood sugar continues to plunge. They then do not feel well. They experience hypoglycaemic (low blood sugar) symptoms such as having cold sweats, shaking and even fainting.

They can feel irritable, cannot function mentally or feel depressed. When their blood sugar is chronically below normal but not low enough to make them faint they can have low moods or feel below par. When they have eaten, especially sugar, they can feel elated and can be boisterous and be their normal selves again quickly.

7) Feeling sleepy after meals

It is possible that the alcohol resulting from fermentation make them feel sleepy. Some people may have a species of Candida which is a more efficient fermenter and therefore more alcohol is produced easily to affect them often. The complaint is often likened to drinking too much alcohol after eating. There are certainly other explanation for the Candida toxins causing sleepiness after meals.

8) Decreased tolerance of alcohol

Many patient have observed that they can't drink as much alcohol as they used to. Even a small amount can make them feel drunk or they suffer a bad hangover effect. If you imagine this scenario: there is already a variable amount of alcohol in the body even before drinking alcohol in those with a Candida problem. The drink that you have contains a further amount of alcohol and sugar. The sugar is then further fermented into alcohol when it gets into the body in patients. So the total amount of alcohol can be more substantial than is realised even though only a small amount of alcohol is intentionally consumed.

9) Weight issue

it is not uncommon for patients to complain that their weight has shot up rapidly over a short period of time. Some even swore that their food intake was minimal and they even exercise regularly but yet the weight had not shifted and their thyroid function (that controls the metabolism in all of us) was normal. I tell those patients that I do not directly deal with weight issues, but their health. If that is improved then the weight will shift as has happened to a number of my patients. Of course the more carbohydrate and calories they put into their body, the more likely they will gain weight and therefore they will always have to be aware of what they put into their body. I feel that the Candida toxins retain fluid—like carrying many 'bags' of small amounts of fluid. With resolution of the problem, the fluid would be released.

10) Recurrent urinary symptoms or increased frequency of micturation

Some patients had bacteria infections in the urinary tract which of course had to be treated appropriately. Quite often they did not have bacteria in the urine on microscopic examination of the urine. Those patients's urinary symptoms cleared when the Candida problem was dealt with.

11) Recurrent vaginal thrush

Over the years I have seen quite a few patients with this problem. My contention is that those patients with this form of vaginal thrush will not be able to stop the recurrence until the Candida problem has been sorted out. Up to 90 percent of vaginal discharge is caused by Candida Albicans and that can easily be treated by your GP using the 'once' treatment of 150mg. of Diflucan orally but if it keeps coming back then the tummy thrush needs to be sorted out before you can expect the vaginal discharge not to recur. Of course other infections can cause vaginal discharge and that must be sorted out if patients do not respond readily to the Candida overgrowth treatment.

Oral thrush is common in babies and older (especially denture-wearing) folks, but it can occur at any age group. It is also caused by overgrowth of Candida Albicans and is treated using the antifungal drugs of Nystatin liquid/lozenges or Amphotericin lozenges. Candida inhabits our gut from the mouth to the end of the gastrointestinal tract at the anus.

Pruritus anus (itchy bottom) is not an uncommon association with the Candida overgrowth. In children worms such as threadworms must be excluded as the worms also cause anal itching and need to be treated differently.

Do not forget that men can also get the equivalent of the female vaginal thrush - penile thrush. This normally occurs in uncircumcised male and especially in those with a weakened immune system.

An often asked question is whether the Candida problem is contagious. It is not. But the above mentioned three conditions can be. Vaginal and penile thrush can be contracted through sexual activity and oropharnygeal thrush through kissing.

12) Skin and nail fungal infections

Very commonly associated with the Candida problem. Whether it is a common symptom that the skin and nails become infected by the fungi or whether it is just a coincidental association, I do not know exactly. It is likely to be related to the Candida overgrowth for I do see that, for example, athlete's foot clears with the usual treatment, when the Candida is treated—though paronychia (fungal infection of the nails) takes much longer to clear; antifungal creams will also need to be used on those sites.

13) Halitosis

Commonly called bad breath. Patients are usually alerted to this condition by their spouses or close friends. Patients have usually been to their dentists to exclude dental decays and to have their oral hygiene checked. They have usually been told that there is nothing untoward in that department but yet the halitosis persist. This is commonly due to fermentation in the gut with the gas rising to the mouth. This condition can be resolved easily by treating the Candida problem.

14) Less common symptoms

These include nausea and vomiting, headaches, muscular aches and pains, and joint pain.

I have had patients whose ankle puffiness was not due to heart conditions. The puffiness disappeared on treatment of the Candida as toxins from the fermentation had caused the patients to retain fluid.

One interesting story that I want to share with you is that of Jackie. She was 12 years old and had always been well until a year prior when she started developing joint pains and swelling of her knuckles. She was diagnosed as suffering from juvenile rheumatoid arthritis by her local specialist. For 9 months she had been on stronger and stronger anti-inflammatory drugs to stop her progressive joint problems. Unfortunately they did not help much. I saw her and tested her and realised that her problem could be related to the dampness and moulds in her house which is 300 years old. Fortunately the parents were in a position to move to a newer built and drier house very quickly. Her pain and the swellings in her hands subsided very soon in the new house and there has been no recurrence of symptoms so far. She did not have tummy symptoms related to Candida but I think it was only a matter of time before they would have emerged if she remained in the mouldy and damp house. Though she had lived in that house ever since she was born she had no symptoms prior to the age of 11. Problems started when she reached puberty and various hormonal changes happened. I am postulating that this was what happened to her to make her intolerant to the moulds. By the way, I have also treated her mother for tummy problems due to Candida, but she has no joint problems and did not react to various moulds that I tested. Her tummy symptoms resolved when the overgrowth was treated. The story is interesting because keeping Jackie away from the moulds and reducing yeast and sugar in her diet has led to her being free from her joint problems, a result that could not be achieved with drugs alone.

Psychiatric manifestations

One 52 year old lady was brought to see me by her family not too long ago. Six months prior to that she had been sectioned (compulsory hospital admission and treatment, by law, without the need for the patient's consent) but was then discharged and was placed on a large quantity of medication for her depression and bizarre mental behaviour. Two months after I had started to treat her Candida, I was persuaded by her family to write a letter to her doctor to have her medication reduced, as the patient was feeling and functioning so much better. At the time of writing this, the pyschiatrist has agreed to see her again to reassess her status and she is awaiting an appointment to see him and still feeling well in herself. The trigger for her bizarre mental symptoms was the intense marital stress she had at that time.

Exaggerated pre-menstrual tension

A less typical problem that I have seen and helped satisfactorily was exaggerated pre-menstrual tension. Amanda aged 35 came to see me for her tummy symptoms of bloating and discomfort, and increasing weight despite her eating very little. She was treated for the Candida overgrowth in the usual way. When I saw her again, a month later, she was happy as she lost some weight and her tummy was free from symptoms. She then said that much to her surprise her pre-menstrual symptoms during her last menstrual cycle were much less severe than usual. Normally a week before her period was due she would feel very tired and irritable. Next day she would become 'manic' shouting at everybody for the slightest reason and her husband described her as 'a raving lunatic'. This sort of behaviour would last till her period started whence she became her usual jolly self again. She had not mentioned the pre-menstrual symptoms as she did not think they were related to her main complaints.

When I saw her for a third time one month later, not only had her presenting symptoms abated, but she had not had any of her usual pre-menstrual symptoms. Since then those symptoms have not reappeared and she is sticking to her sugar-free diet unwaveringly and taking the antifungal herbs when she deemed necessary.

Peri-menopausal symptoms

Katherine aged 51 presented with symptoms of tummy bloating and tiredness. When her Candida problem was treated, not only did her original symptoms become better but also her menopausal symptoms of hot flushes and sweating became much less. The condition stayed that way as long as she did not have too much sugar. When she overdosed on sugar the hot flushes came back and then she had to avoid sugar totally for a while to get back to normal. Again those symptoms were not mentioned in the original discussion as she accepted that, at her age, having menopausal symptoms was normal. It was not the Candida overgrowth that was responsible for her perimenopausal condition but the overgrowth was linked to the intensity of her symptoms.

In the above cases the Candida was triggered by the patient's fluctuating hormone levels. Note also that the Candida problem can exacerbate existing conditions that arise from those hormonal changes.

Christina's letter

I include what Christina has written in her letter to me. She described many typical symptoms and some triggering factors. She has given me permission to show it as she wants people to be aware of the various states of health that one may go through with a Candida problem. Though it is reproduced here in the third person, it was written by her about her.

Christina, now 39 years old, had unknowingly suffered from Candida for most of her life. She always felt tired, struggled to get up in the mornings, was very fussy about what she ate but she ate a lot of what she liked (mainly carbohydrates), found it impossible to put on weight and could be quite irritable and stroppy.

As a child she was picked on at school for being so thin but as an adult felt quite happy that she could eat large quantities of what she liked and didn't put on weight.

Most days she would have bags under her eyes also known as allergy shiners! These were always really exaggerated when she contracted childhood illnesses such as chickenpox.

In her twenties she used to go night clubbing regularly but could not tolerate alcohol. However, drinking the full sugar varieties of lemonade/coke or Pepsi used to give a real high, to the point where strangers would ask what she was 'taking'! (Now known to be her own little fermentation factory in her gut which turned the sugar to ethanol!)

Skiing always relieved her symptoms as she had lots of energy and really felt alive but thought it was the enjoyment of the skiing rather than the relief high altitude made to her symptoms.

Christina always seemed to have clogged up sinuses which were not problematic except when she went out for a walk or cycle ride as she had to make sure she had a tissue at the ready and as a child got told off regularly for picking her nose! She would be bloated after eating which created 'itchy bits' where the skin constantly stretched and contracted just above her hips. Sometimes she would get a very itchy back too and would often get pussy spots and boils like her body was trying to get rid of something toxic.

When she was in her early twenties she contracted bronchitis abroad on holiday which was treated in hospital for 5 days with really strong antibiotics. The day after arriving home she had what was thought to be food poisoning and was in hospital for a further 5 days with severe diarrhoea and vomiting. However, this may not have been food poisoning but the effects of the antibiotics

Since this Christina suffered with IBS and her aches and pains, tiredness and irritability gradually got worse especially when she was hungry. However, it was still manageable so she never sought to get a diagnosis as she didn't like going to the doctor. She also craved bread, in actual fact was addicted to it, and ate 2-4 slices at least twice a day. (For some reason your mind will often crave the very thing which is causing the biggest issue.)

Bloating after eating was just part of daily living, clothes put on in the morning would become tight and restrictive after lunch so would regularly cause mild stomach cramps and a frequent need to stool. Damp days would really make her feel low and were a real energy zapper. Visiting old damp buildings such as an old watermill would trigger those annoying stomach cramps within 20 minutes.

Candida also meant that sexual intercourse was often painful and generally not the pleasurable experience it should be.

However, in January 2007 a strange sequence of events changed everything. Christina's IBS symptoms had been getting a lot worse in the lead up to Christmas but she put this down eating rich food and stress at work. After Christmas she contracted a cold but thought nothing of and still went in to work but during December they had been replacing the carpet tiles in her office.

These events lead Christina to contract leaky gut syndrome. It was the scariest experience of her life as she was losing ¼ stone per week whilst eating more than usual but constant diarrhoea meant she wasn't getting enough nourishment and thought she was going to die.

Unfortunately, due to her lack of previous visits to the doctors about her symptoms the doctors made the assumption she had an eating disorder and as her mind did not have enough fuel to function properly she could not convey the true problems.

Christina was latterly diagnosed with post-traumatic stress disorder which the leaky gut syndrome had triggered together with severe depression which she had therapy for but she knew no amount of therapy was going to clear the fog which had been left behind in her head.

Her IBS was extreme, she was malnourished and weak, days were planned around where toilets were and the tiredness was indescribable (it was like daily living with a stomach bug). She felt trapped, despair and that there was no way out or proper help. All this led to her taking an overdose (which was thankfully unsuccessful!)

It was the dietician she was under at the time who started her on the track of Candida. Christina was asked to try removing sugar and yeast from her diet as she had already removed wheat and dairy. This helped. Her IBS attacks were reduced to 3-5 times a week and her mood lifted a little but she was still eating carbohydrates.

Daily living was difficult, like having a physical disability that no one could see and Christina lived in constant fear of getting a cold, flu or stomach bug as she was so thin and had no reserves to be able to resist such an illness.

The biggest help came when she was referred to an Allergist.

Initial tests showed Small Intestinal Bactria Overgrowth (SIBO) and gut fermentation, the formal diagnosis for probable Candida. Her gut fermentation levels were extreme, so explained why she was unable to beat her depression, as it is one of the symptoms of Candida and allergies.

Antibiotics were used to treat the SIBO but made her more foggy headed and depressed for a while as antibiotics increase the gut fermentation. Strong freeze-dried probiotics were also tried but they unfortunately exacerbated her symptoms.

Nystatin powder, an antifungal, was prescribed which significantly helped manage the IBS symptoms of bloating, aching joints. But the foggy head, depression and extreme tiredness were still there.

The next revelation came from skin testing. She found she had numerous chemical and food sensitivities, including formaldehyde and Candida.

She now had an answer as to what triggered her leaky gut symptoms because formaldehyde is in new carpets (amongst a lot of other things such as air fresheners and perfumes). Previously she had always assumed it was something she was eating which had caused extreme IBS but the formaldehyde in the carpets together with the cold virus was her tipping point.

Following the second session of skin testing Christina was advised to restrict her diet to only the foods she had been tested for as she was given neutralisation vaccines for these which were taken every day. Neutralisation vaccines are a small sample of the tested item which is watered down to a level which can be best tolerated.

Her diet consisted of meats, fish and vegetables low in

sugar on a four day rotation basis (caveman diet). Although she really struggled the first week as the craving for carbohydrates was immense, the effects by the beginning of the second week were truly amazing. The foggy head completely cleared and it felt like she had emerged from the dark and transformed into feeling like a proper human again. Life was no longer based on fear of where the toilet was as IBS attacks were reduced to rare occasions.

Whilst on this restricted diet Christina identified that plugin air fresheners were a trigger, not just food. This was a big surprise as she had previously spent countless times analysing and wondering what it was that she had eaten that caused each upset. Even specialists had said work out what you are eating and cut it out but these personal trials just lead to a fear of many foods and an unbalanced diet. The problem then remained of how to avoid scents and chemicals in today's modern world. All things in her own home were replaced with scent free and organic products which helped a lot, but people's aftershave and perfume at work were unavoidable.

So although Christina had significantly improved, after nearly a year on this diet she started feeling trapped again. The diet controlled her Candida but it did not treat it. Her friendships had suffered as she found it difficult to eat out socially and her medication and diet of organic meat, fish and vegetables was very expensive.

This quickly changed after the recommendation to see Dr Choy.

Simple tests were performed which on first visit confirmed that formaldehyde and Candida were Christina's biggest allergens and she was given treatment.

Within six weeks of treatment with a neutralising vaccine and dietary supplements, she stopped taking Nystatin powder and had started introducing new foods to her diet including carbohydrates.

The biggest improvements for Christina are that her energy has returned, she is waking up early and feeling refreshed, her weight is steadily increasing which has boosted her confidence.

Most importantly, she feels that she has a future to look forward to.

Christina's case history shows what the Candida problem can do to a person and how when dealt with, it can literally change a person's life.

Doctors are not taught about the Candida problem at medical school. We only know about Candida for its association with vaginal thrush, oropharngeal thrush and fungal infections of the skin and nails. So it is little wonder that when patients mention Candida to their doctor as a possible cause of their symptoms, they are laughed at or the notion is dismissed outright.

4

DIET

AN UNDERSTANDING OF THE ROLE OF DIET

My approach is very simple and straighforward and all my patients can stick to it. The initial reaction of some patients is that they cannot give up sugar as they are addicted to it, but they all do it. Some cannot do it immediately because the Candida problem affected their sugar level regulation. These people can have their blood sugar level come crashing down making them feel very unwell, and they need sugary things to bring their blood sugar level up to prevent them from collapsing. Therefore I consider it cruel or unsympathetic to insist avoiding sugars strictly when they have this problem. This phenomenon will come under control when the Candida problem is treated and then they can be advised to adhere to their diet more rigorously. They are then in a position to do it well. In fact some of them have remarked when I see them subsequently that they cannot stand the taste of chocolate or sweets since their recovery and do not ever want to eat them again.

We eat things for two main reasons. One is because we just want to eat them. We can always not want to eat them as that is within our control. Second is we need to eat them, because when the blood sugar is down it makes us feel unwell—we cannot say we don't want to eat them: we just collapse. This situation is not within our control. However, when the Candida is being treated, we can gradually convert the 'need to' to 'want to' which is within our control. Remember that it is important not to create another problem whilst treating the existing problem.

Most of the information available from books, internet or practitioners will state that you have to avoid all yeasty foods, wheat, milk and coffee as well as other foods for all kinds of reasons. Whilst they may have their own reasons for saying that, I find that in the vast majority of patients, there is no necessity to do it unless they are also sensitive to those foods. A great deal of what needs to be done in terms of diet initially depends on the patient's medical history. Very few patients can follow a strict diet for long, but those patients that are very ill or who have lots of symptoms will do it initially. When they feel slightly better they begin to resent the fact that they have to be on such a restricted diet which hampers their lives in order to feel better. I have met patients who have been on a very restricted diet for more than twenty years and they have not felt that much better. I therefore assume that the foods that they have avoided cannot account for all their medical complaints—the diet has just made them feel miserable. They felt less unwell but the symptoms were still present and they had not recovered.

With the Candida problem, patients can get what I term a secondary food intolerance which will abate when the Candida problem is sorted out, unless there is a primary intolerance to those foods. By that I mean that all kinds of foods seem to give them symptoms. Others would use the term 'leaky' gut which denotes that food molecules of different sizes get through the gut wall (which shouldn't normally happen) to set up food allergic symptoms to explain their symptoms. As I have said before—and it is important for me to repeat it and I make no apologies for continuously saying it—I liken the effect (not the 'leaky' gut) to a wound on your skin: any particle that falls into the wound is going to hurt or irritate you. You may think it is the particle that causes the problem, but when the wound is healed that same particle will not hurt you. You can prevent things from falling into the wound so that you are not hurt, but the wound is still there when not treated. You will feel less bad, but you are not better—the problem is still there.

Nevertheless it is wise to refrain from eating something that you know is going to hurt you, at least for a while until things are better. Then you can reintroduce those foods gradually and you will be pleased to find that you can tolerate them. There has been some research on Candida-induced late onset gluten sensitivity. Avoiding gluten-containing products do make them feel better because gluten sensitivity can also give rise to symptoms of abdominal bloating, pain and diarrhoea. In those patients I believe the gluten sensitivity is secondary to the Candida problem and can abate when the Candida problem is sorted. Do note that in the majority of patients with the Candida problem the problem did not occur because they have been eating badly, but because eating sugar when the Candida problem is there will make you feel much worse. In fact, in the patients that I have seen over many years, in the great majority this problem was not due to them eating badly (which triggered off the problem).

My experience is based on 35 years of feedback from patients and therefore I may express different views to others who have not dealt with patients with this problem for as long as I have. Almost everything that we eat commonly contains or breaks down into sugar in the gut, and so anything can seem to give rise to symptoms by feeding the Candida and causing fermentation. Wheat is a carbohydrate which breaks down into sugar, milk contains lactose (milk sugar) which can cause symptoms.

Avoiding these foods by themselves is not going to resolve the problem, though it can make patients feel less bad and therefore better than when they were eating those 'wrong' foods. Some foods can give rise to symptoms fairly quickly and so you can establish the correlation easily, whilst other foods may take a longer time for symptoms to come on and therefore it is so much more difficult to see the association. The thing is not to eat the foods that you know are going to give you symptoms till your Candida problem is sorted out—even though those foods are not the underlying cause of your problems.

Following a very strict diet is difficult especially for those who have to lead an active social life. I liken the diet problem again to a wound you have on your body: if you scratch it, it will hurt you. If you do not scratch it you are not going to make it hurt more, but the wound is still there and needs other treatment to get it better quickly. You apply things to it to make it heal. When the wound is healed, touching or scratching it lightly is not going to hurt. So wait till the Candida is better before reintroducing larger amounts of the offending foods even though, as I have said before, they may not be the direct cause of your Candida overgrowth.

Experience shows me that fewer than 10 percent of patients with Candida problems also have a yeast intolerance, and far fewer than that have wheat or milk intolerance (this is not a scientific fact but just based on my own observations). Patients with other primary food allergies also have to avoid those relevant foods in order to get full resolution of their problems. With my patients I can test if other foods are causing problems. Self-diagnosis is much more difficult—it has to be on a trial and error basis. But sugar is by far the most important and relevant thing to avoid.

My advice to these patients is to avoid sugar in the form of chocolate, all the sweet foods such as sweets, puddings, cakes, biscuits, sweet drinks etc. Cut out honey, syrup and dried fruits. All fresh fruits contain fruit sugar but some have more and these fruits can give symptoms even when eaten in small amounts. Avoid grapes, melons, bananas, mangoes and papayas. Other fruits when eaten in larger amounts will also give rise to symptoms but in general most of my patients can tolerate some of the other fruits. With fruit juices, it is best to avoid them or have very little amounts. Avoid wine or beer: it is not so much the alcohol but the sugar in them which is the problem. Other alcohol such as spirits and champagne seem to be better tolerated. Sweet wine is sweet because it contains more sugar. If you drink spirits, take them neat or with water. If a mixer is used, make sure it is sugar free.

Do remember that dried fruits such as figs and dates contain a lot of natural sugar and so should be avoided.

Doctors who advocate a yeast free diet as well in the treatment of Candida are more concerned about the reactions to the Candida antigens. An antigen is a foreign protein which when in your body can cause an allergic reaction. It is reckoned that there are at least 70 yeast antigens. By keeping to a yeast free diet, you can at least reduce added exposure to yeast antigens. As stated my observations over the years have led me to believe that this is not a big issue in most of the patients that I had seen.

Food for thought in the literal sense: we have been eating foods for years and people throughout the world eat more or less the same foods though they may prepare them differently. If the foods are indeed the primary cause of the Candida problem then almost everybody would be suffering from it. There is no doubt that the world has changed dramatically especially over the last fifty years. Factors that trigger the Candida problem were not there or were present less frequently: now they are an everyday occurrence. Therefore the incidence of the Candida problem is greater now and awareness of this possibility is on the rise.

Sugary foods aggravate the situation when the Candida is already in a state of imbalance, but not otherwise. This I have to emphasise as I do not believe that sugar is the cause of the Candida problem. It is just prudent not to eat sugar whilst the Candida is being treated—not to mention that sugar is associated with other health problems. There are many factors in life which can cause an imbalance of the Candida. As it is impossible to know if your Candida is in a state of imbalance without waiting for symptoms to appear first, it is best not to eat too much (or avoid) sugar. Health practitioners rightly advise the reduction of sugar because of its link to so many other health issues.

Almost all my patients go back to eating some of the 'wrong' foods. It is the amount that they have to be careful with, and that varies with the individual. Some patients tolerate more, others less. It is not a diet for life but rather a style of life. You choose not to eat sugary things in your daily life but you should be able to cope with them, such as when you are invited for dinner and not wanting to make a fuss about what you are being served (when you are better). If you have more than what your body can cope with at that time, you may have symptoms but at least you know what you have done. It is not just a question of having symptoms, but of knowing what caused your symptoms. If you do not want the symptoms just do not eat so much of the food, or avoid it for a while if it gives you symptoms. Maybe the amount you were eating was too much for your body to cope with efficiently—reducing the quantity may be sufficient to avoid symptoms. Or you may need to avoid that particular food for a period of time before trying it again.

Patients with digestive enzyme deficiency problems, such as that in Coeliac disease where the enzyme for digesting gluten (found in most grains) is absent or is present but in inadequate amounts, can never eat those foods without getting disagreeable symptoms. This is the case in those with primary gluten sensitivity. But there are various enzymes that are available commercially which may help to tolerate small amounts of the 'disagreeable' foods. Some research has suggested that Candida may trigger the Coeliac condition. It is too early to know if that conclusion is true. The same also applies to those with lactose deficiency (they cannot digest milk sugar-lactose). Milk and milk products can give them tummy aches and diarrhoea. Some may get away with lactose-free milk. These two conditions are the most common enzyme deficiently states, and tests can be done to confirm the existence of these conditions.

We have to be aware that even though wheat and milk can give rise to symptoms in Candida patients, they should cease to be a problem once the Candida problem has been resolved, provided the condition is not due to enzyme deficiency. If they continue to cause problems then the above-mentioned conditions need to be looked into; for any other medical condition can exist alongside a Candida problem. The fact that you have a Candida problem does not mean you cannot have something else as well.

5

DIAGNOSIS

A WAY TO DIAGNOSE THE PROBLEM

When I was a medical student in Singapore, some forty plus years ago, the one thing that was continuously drummed into us was the importance of history taking. That accounts for 70 percent of the information needed to get a correct diagnosis. If the practitioner listens carefully and asks the right questions then one can come to the right diagnosis easily. This is never more true than with the diagnosis of Candida overgrowth. Very often the patient gives 'pointers' towards the diagnosis and the answers to the right questions then support it. I always believe that patients' observations are always correct unless we strongly suspect them of malingering. Their interpretation of those events however may not be what they thought it was. For example many patients say that when they eat bread or pasta,or drink milk, they get symptoms. So they avoid those foods and say that they are 'allergic' to them. If other foods also affected them, then those foods were also avoided; so their diet became very restricted. But their symptoms remained and persisted despite their very rigid diet. It is like painting yourself into a

54

---

[1] The National Science Foundation

corner: you cannot get out without stepping over the paint. So there must be other reasons to account for their persistent symptoms. As I have stated earlier, Candida fermentation can account for the symptoms they suffer with those foods.

Conventional tests such as blood tests, various types of X-ray examinations and endoscopies are important and relevant. If the various tests are normal, it is good to know what you haven't got. The doctors can rule out and tell you that you haven't got any sinister problem though they may not be able to tell you exactly what is causing your symptoms.

There are several tests for Candida. These include the detection of Candida antibodies in BLOOD, SALIVA and URINE. By itself the presence of antibodies to Candida antigens does not indicate a Candida overgrowth. The prescence of Candida in stools (faeces) has also been used and again that does not indicate a Candida imbalance.

Gut Fermentation Test

This measures the alcohol level in the blood after drinking a standard dose of sugar in a drink. If the alcohol level is above a certain level, it indicates that there is fermentation. Although the Candida species are the most common organism to ferment sugar in the gut, bacteria can also cause fermentation. This however is a useful test to have and alongside the history it can support the diagnosis.

Sometimes if fermentation occurs further down the gut such as in the large intestine the test may not pick this up and can therefore be negative.

Muscle Testing

This is an unorthodox method of testing and seemingly unscientific but nevertheless invaluable and appropriate. It must be realised that methods are scientific only when they have been investigated and declared by the investigative body to work according to known scientific principles. If no research has been done into those methods then they may be unorthodox, but they cannot be deemed unscientific.

Muscle testing is very simple. No equipment is needed and certainly no needles. The patient stands facing me with one outstretched arm—usually the stronger right arm in most cases. The outstretched arm is pressed downwards by me to assess the muscle tone—it should stay up if done properly. The patient then holds on to a tube of normal saline (body's own salt solution) with the other hand and, when pressed down again by me the outstretched arm should still stay up. This is the control—to check the muscle tone when holding onto something that is not incompatible with the patient. Next with the same pose the patient now holds on to a tube containing extract of Candida Albicans and if that is incompatible with them the outstretched right arm weakens and comes down when pressed. This confirms a diagnosis of Candida overgrowth for me. Variants of this method are being used by other practitioners for different purposes. It is not just the muscle testing but the interpretation of it together with the clinical history that leads one to strongly suspect whether there is a Candida problem. The subsequent management must lead to an improvement in the medical complaints if you are correct in your assessment of the symptoms.

This phenomenon was first noted by Dr. Goodheart , an American chiropractor in the mid 1960s. He noted that in certain of his patients with medical disorders particular muscles felt weakened when he examined them. In time it was noted that certain muscles correlate with the pathway of certain meridians. Meridians according to Chinese Traditional Medicine are pathways for the flow of energy in the body. If the meridians are blocked they indicate that there is a medical disorder and the associated muscle will be weakened on examination. The importance of energy flow is a very important concept in Traditional Chinese Medicine which has been practised for more than four thousand years. I have to emphasise that what I do has not the remotest link to Traditional Chinese Medicine and I do not practice it.

Over the years various doctors have written about this phenomenon and have adapted this technique to help them do other things. I only use this technique to check for various incompatibilities. This technique is at least as reliable and is arguably more appropriate than the standard method of skin or blood tests which can often show false positive or false negative readings. A false positive result occurs when the test shows a reading that is positive even though the patient knows that the substance indicated does not affect him. A false negative is when a thing that the patient or the practitioner strongly suspects affects the patient does not show a positive result on testing. So sometimes it is difficult to interpret the test, and even if it is a true positive test it does not necessarily mean that is the root cause of their symptoms. It just means that the item/items in question is not right for the body. For example, if a patient with rhinorrhea (runny nose) presents in the winter months, and the skin prick test showed a positive reaction to grass pollen, it does not mean that the pollen is the underlying reason for the symptom (in winter), for there is no grass pollen in the air in winter in the Northern hemisphere.

With the muscle testing I can also test to see if other things affect the patients as well. In this way I can advise the patients appropriately. There is no need to avoid foods that do not directly help them to be better.

Some years ago I was asked by a member of the House of Lords to appear before a Select Committe to support muscle testing as a method of testing for allergies. I turned down the invitation as muscle testing is not a way of testing for allergies. Allergy is associated with a raised level of a class of antibody called Ig E though it is recognised that there are some allergic reactions that are not Ig E linked. This antibody can only be detected on blood examination, and muscle testing does not involve blood testing and therefore cannot determine the level of Ig E.

Muscle testing is however a very good and practical way of seeing what is not right for a person. To the lay person the term allergy is used to convey an incompatible item causing various degrees of unwarranted clinical reactions. However to doctors it means a very specific clinical phenomenon associated with certain changes in the blood which can usually be noted. Hence a lot of doctors become very irritated when patients tell them that they are allergic to various foods. The proper term to use is 'adverse reaction' to the foods as this term would include allergy as one of the causes of an adverse reaction.

Stool Examination

Has also been used but the critics would say that the presence of Candida in the stool does not indicate Candida overgrowth, as Candida is present in the gut normally. This is true and so this test does not really help. Vaginal thrush does not equate to a Candida overgrowth in the gut and excessive Candida in the vagina can be confirmed with a high vaginal swab for subsequent examination and culture. There are lots of patients who present with a Candida problem but who have no history and no symptoms of vaginal thrush.

Saliva Test

This is a simple test though the validity of this test is questioned. Spit into a glass of water first thing in the morning before brushing your teeth. If you have Candida then after 20 minutes you will see filaments dangling from the spit to the bottom of the glass; there may even be a layer of 'debris'at the bottom of the glass. If that does not happen then it is said there is no overgrowth of Candida in the gut.

As you can gather by now there is no reliable scientific test for a Candida overgrowth and therefore taking a full and clear history and asking the right questions remain the most important diagnostic tools. Some doctors use a questionnaire listing the symptoms of Candida overgrowth and sensitivity to environmental yeasts to help them confirm the diagnosis. When the treatment also leads to the patient feeling better and to disappearance of symptoms, then the correlation is certainly there even though there may not be any scientifically accredited test to confirm such a correlation. To the patients, getting a diagnosis and feeling better with the right treatment is the most important thing. They are not concerned with any academic debate about the best method for diagnosing Candida. They just want to be better!

It is of utmost importance to realise that a positive on any tests does not necessarily mean that the item is the reason for the problem, and taking steps to counter it may not necessarily lead to improvement. It just means that the item tested is not compatible with the person. Example: if you have rhinitis (runny nose) in the winter and skin prick tests showed a large reaction to grass pollen, it can safely be concluded that grass pollen is not the cause of your complaint, for there is no grass pollination in the winter.

6

TREATMENT

A SIMPLE AND EFFECTIVE WAY OF TREATMENT

The aim of treatment is to restore the balance of Candida in the gut. You cannot get rid of Candida from your body totally because it is a normal inhabitant in the body. Unlike bacteria from an infection which are foreign to your body and which should be got rid of, Candida is part of you. You strive to get back the balance. There are two important prongs of treatment:

1) reducing the Candida overgrowth
2) re-establishing the balance of the gut micro-organisms

1A) REDUCING THE AMOUNT OF CANDIDA

You can use conventional drugs (antifungals), however these do have side effects some of which can be severe. For example when using the antifungal Nizoral you are advised to monitor your liver function regularly through blood tests. Though the drug can be effective in reducing the Candida levels, it may also harm the liver. A drug which I have used regularly in the past is Nystatin. It is supposedly harmless and

I did not encounter any reported side effects. Unfortunately this drug is now not readily available in most chemists in this country, though Nystatin powder is still available via a specialised supplier. But a lot of my patient prefer a non-drug antifungal.

I have used a non drug (herbal) antifungal which has proven effective over the last twenty more years: Caprilic Plus. It is a combination of various natural (herbal) antifungals which do not have any known side effects. When the Candida is killed off, you may experience the 'die off' effect, which is caused when toxins from the dying Candida are released. This does not happen to everybody who takes this antifungal and is not a side effect. Even when patients get the 'die off' effect the symptoms do not last long. With some patients who experience the 'die off' symptoms with resultant adverse symptoms which are severe, I stop the antifungal for a few days till the symptoms subside and then resume with a lower dosage before gradually increasing the dose back to the original prescribed dose and this generally solves the problem of the 'die off'. The 'die off' is normally just an exaggeration of the Candida symptoms and lasts 2 to 3 days and is not dangerous. Though most patients cope with the standard dose, each of us is different and may need a different dose regime. You always have to find the balance of getting the patient better quicker and the degree of 'die off' symptoms.

Caprilic Plus

This is a combination of various natural antifungals which I have devised with a colleague of mine, after having used various types of natural antifungals. Each herbal antifungal does yield a certain percentage of response but not everybody will respond. I use a combination of herbal antifungal as I get a greater response. This combination has proved very useful to me in its effectiveness as an antifungal over the last thirty or more years. Below I have listed briefly the rationale for its use based on the research of others. I have also included here a brief summary of each of the ingredients of Caprilic Plus.

1) *Caprilic Acid* inhibits the growth of Candida Albicans and other detrimental fungi in the intestine. It is incorporated into the cell membrane of the yeast (fungi) thereby causing rupture and killing the cell.

2) *Pau D'Arco* kills/suppresses detrimental microbes in the gut due to its napthoquinone content. It is also thought to be useful in the treatment of some types of intestinal parasites, viruses and even in the treatment of malaria (due to its lapachol content).

3) *Garlic* enhances the growth of some beneficial bacteria such as the Bifidobacter and the Lactobaccillus group. It is also helpful in the treatment of salmonella, shigella and the helicobacter pylori.

4) *Aloe Vera* inhibits various types of detrimental bacteria and fungi including Candida Albicans and the Trichophyton species.

5) *Grapefruit Seed Extract* kills/suppresses many types of detrimental microorganisms in the gut including Candida Albicans, Aspergillus and Trichophyton species.

6) *Cinnamon* inhibits the growth of Candida and other forms of detrimental fungi and bacteria. It alleviates flatulence and exerts antihelminthic (treatment for worms) activity against ascaris (roundworm).

7) *Peppermint* improves the function of many aspects of the digestive system, and alleviates diarrhoea and flatulence.

8) *Slippery Elm* alleviates diarrhoea and some symptoms of acidity.

9) *Lemon Grass* inhibits growth of Candida. Besides it's many other useful functions on the body, it calms the nervous system and has benefits for the skin.

10) *Glutamine* is an essential 'fuel' for the villi cells (concerned with absorption of nutrients) of the intestinal wall and it strongly enhances the health of the digestive system, and ability of the neutrophil cells of the immune system to destroy detrimental bacteria. It can also alleviate carbohydrate cravings and elevated blood sugar levels.

I would start the treatment with one capsule of the Caprilic Plus twice or three times a day to be taken at meal times, depending on the severity and types of symptoms the patients present with. After three weeks I would normally continue with one capsule twice a day for a further four weeks, or up the dose depending on the response. Then I either advise a further course of the Caprilic Plus for four weeks or change the patient over to a good probiotic. Depending on my assessment of the patient, if I feel there is going to be much 'die off' reaction, I might start with just one capsule a day till I see them again. It is impossible to list the criteria to determine the appropriate starting dose. That can only be acquired with experience.

Various non drug anti-fungals are being used and have been successful in the treatment of Candida but I must say that not every patient will respond to any single herb or drug. The combination of herbs in Caprilic Plus seems to give a much better response rate, which I have observed, having been using it for the last 30+ years.

'Die-off' reaction

This sometimes occurs when patients with Candida are treated with antifungals. This can manifest as an exaggeration of their Candida symptoms or simply feeling 'fluey' or having more frequent bowel movements—the body's attempt to get rid of the Candida toxin. This does not usually happen with the Caprillic Plus that I use and if it does occur and the patient cannot cope with the symptoms then I stop the antifungal for a day or two and wait till the symptoms subside before restarting the antifungal—this has always resolved the problem.

I see this less commonly with herbal antifungals than with drug antifungals such as Amphotericine or other more powerful drug antifungals. Some people liken this to what is not uncommonly seen in conventional medicine and is known as the 'Herxheimer' reaction caused by the organisms being killed off and their toxins being released into the body faster than the body can handle them. Herxheimer first reported this phenomenon towards the end of the nineteenth century when he was treating Syphilis with mercury. Patients felt worse initially with symptoms of fever, joint aches and other symptoms.

This was ascribed to the spirochetes (organisms causing Syphilis) being killed and toxins released. Subsequently other drugs like antifungals and antibiotics used in treatment of other diseases were also noted to have this reaction especially in the treatment of Lymes Disease (a disease transmitted by ticks and caused by the Borrelia bacteria). This reaction, if it occurs using Caprillic Plus, is not serious and last usually for just a couple of days, though it may last longer in some people. Some people refer to this as the 'healing crisis' and generally patients improve or get well after this. Majority of patients do not need to go through this 'healing crisis' in order to get better.

1B) NOT FEEDING THE CANDIDA

The idea is not to feed the Candida whilst things are being done to redress the Candida imbalance. In my experience foods are often not the cause of the patient's Candida problem. Certain foods can aggravate the condition until it is sorted out but I always advise a reduction of sugar or very sweet foods, or if possible to avoid totally.

When I first encountered the problem, I used to put my patients on a very strict and restricted diet regime. For all kinds of reasons a few patients could not adhere to it. One told me she was in public relations and her job was to entertain corporate clients at every lunchtime and so could not follow her dietary regime as she had to eat and drink alcohol with the clients. Other patients told me similar stories. Surprisingly they all got better even though they had not been able to follow the dietary regime strictly. Over the years I was swayed to thinking about the importance of diets. Though the diet is relevant to getting better, perhaps too much importance had been focused on it. Latterly I had been much relaxed on the diet except the sugar. With children I do not insist on any kind of dietary regime except to avoid sugar as best as possible and I am pleased with the positive response from patients. Many of my patients go back to eating some of the 'wrong foods' when they are better. I tell them that it is not a diet for life but rather a life style. You choose not to eat the 'wrong foods' regularly in your everyday life but you can eat and tolerate them when you have to, when you are better (just like some people choose not to eat meat and become a vegetarian, for religious or other reasons). This is attested to by the feedbacks I have received from patients over the years. When a person chooses to avoid certain foods there is no stress because it is a choice, but when you are being told to avoid certain foods, after a while you can resent it as you have no choice. Therefore it is adopting the right psychological attitude that will make the difference in you being happy or not in following a dietary regime.

Some patients feel very guilty about foods as they think their problem arises because of their poor eating habits. The wrong foods may make their symptoms worse, but if the Candida was already in a state of imbalance triggered by other factors the wrong foods just made them feel worse.

In some patients the Candida toxins affect the regulation of their blood sugar—so that their moods or physical self fluctuate very abruptly. They can feel good and then shortly after they feel lousy—weak, sweaty and can even faint because their blood sugar plunges. So they have to eat sugar to feel better quickly. This cycle is then repeated so they become addicted to foods especially sugar. Under such circumstances it is not right to get them to avoid sugar at all costs, for if they do not get the blood sugar up they will faint. We eat because of two main reasons. First, because we want to eat—like if we are offered chocolate, we can say we don't want as the 'want' is within our control. Second we need to eat as the blood sugar is plunging. The 'need' is not within our control. So the insistence of avoiding sugar in those situations shows that we do not completely understand the problem that the patients are facing. When the Candida problem comes under better control, then the 'need' is converted back to the 'want'. It is then up to the individual patient to resist the 'want'. Most patients can then succeed in controlling the sugar craving and feel much happier for that.

Often patients feel better on a gluten-free diet though some symptoms still persist. When gluten is reintroduced they feel bad. This then leads to a diagnosis of gluten intolerance—understandably. It should be noted that the cell wall of the Candida contain a sequence of amino acids that is the same as that in the gliadin faction of gluten that cause gluten intolerance and when the Candida is in a state of imbalance those amino acids can be triggered. Perhaps that is why patients made the connection between gluten and some of their symptoms. In Coeliac primary disease, which is where there are absent or inadequate gluten enzymes, the avoidance of gluten-containing foods is for life. In secondary gluten intolerance which occurs when the Candida is imbalanced, then when the Candida problem is sorted out, they can tolerate gluten-containing foods again as reported by many of my patients.

Some patients's Candida problems are made worse by damp weather conditions or by visits to damp or mouldy environments. They may be allergic to the fungi in the environment. If the symptoms are significant and do not improve when the Candida imbalance is sorted out, then they need to see a practitioner who can deal with this particular problem. This is exemplified in the case of Vicky.

Vicky was then a 43 year old lady who had a long history of adverse reactions to various foods. She would feel unwell, low energy, generalised rashes, chest and knee pain and other minor symptoms besides tummy bloating and a sluggish bowel. Over the years she had various investigations which turned out negative. A few years ago she was diagnosed as having a Candida problem in Paris (where she was based then) and treated, but her symptoms persisted. When I saw her I also thought that she had a Candida problem and that problem was duly treated by me. Gradually she was able to eat more foods without getting reactions. Her energy improved and her tummy became flat and her bowel function was back to normal. She stayed so well that she went on a trip to Africa and successfully climbed the Uhuru peak of Mount Kilimanjaro with others. She remained well till the start of autumn. Foods gradually began to give her problems again, though nowhere as bad as before. I did several other tests and prescribed her other nutrients. That also did not alleviate the problem. By then the environment was very damp and so I started giving her neutralising treatment for the moulds (fungi) in the environment that she tested positive to. When I saw her again a few weeks later she was able to report that she was feeling better and could cope with foods without any reactions. A few more weeks later she was able to declare herself fit again and tolerating foods. Now she realised why she always felt worse in autumn and the winter months since coming to England 4 years ago.

This indicates the relevance of the environmental moulds in some people with the Candida problem.

Water

It is estimated that between 60% to 70% of our body weight is water. It is as high as 79% in newborn infants. Thirst is a symptom that the body needs water but many people have learned to ignore this symptom and instead have misinterpreted it as being hungry, thereby eating instead and hence making the situation worse. Extreme thirst is definitely a symptom of extreme dehydration and you have to quench the thirst in order for the body to function normally again.

Water has many functions and health benefits for the body besides quenching the thirst. It dissolves waste and toxic substances in the blood and carries them to the kidneys where they are filtered and eliminated. In everyday life your body has to get rid of urea, uric acid and lactic acid as well as waste products from the body's other metabolic processes.

When you are on treatment to get rid of the excess Candida toxins from your body, it is imperative that you drink enough water so that the body can clear the dead Candida and toxins.

The human body also depends on water for its survival. Besides dissolving and carrying the unwanted substances away it is also important for other functions. The brain which is only 1% to 2% of the body weight has about 5% of the blood flow and is comprised of 70% water. If you are dehydrated you can expect your brain to function poorly.

Water is also essential to the synovial fluid in your joints so that they can function smoothly at all times. Dehydration can give rise to joint pains and dysfunction (poor function) of joints.

Water is also important to make your faeces soft so that bowel movements become smooth. Otherwise the faeces can become hard and bowel movement sluggish and painful due to having to strain the body in order to get the bowels functioning.

Water has also been referred to as having antihistamine function but I would personally get a proprietary antihistamine if I need to use it.

Vitamin and Mineral Supplements

Supplements do not directly bring the Candida under control but they do make the body function better thereby responding more readily to the treatment. Deficiencies of various nutrients can lead to the body functioning less efficiently and therefore patients cope with the Candida imbalance and its various symptoms less well. They may also fail to respond to the Candida treatment as well as they could. I do not prescribe lots of supplements but I find that many patients are deficient in Zinc and Magnesium. Other nutrients which are required will depend on the patient's nutritional status and symptoms arising from those deficiencies. These need to be treated at the same time as the treatment for the Candida.

As this book is not about the functions of various nutrients in our body they will not be discussed except for a couple of nutrients which I have found to be of great relevance to Candida imbalances. Zinc is very important to the immune system. When the body is under stress—and stress is not just mental or emotional but can be physical such as working too hard or running around here and there, or fighting any infection—a lot of Zinc is used. Therefore there is less for the immune system. It is not uncommon for a lot of people's symptoms to get worse when they are under stress, thus leading to a lot of doctors saying that the symptoms are due to stress alone. Stress may have triggered off the symptoms but often it is not the underlying cause. Zinc is also important for the skin, hair, nails, joints, libido, and hundreds of metabolic functions in the body. Hence, those systems also suffer to a varying extent when the Zinc level is low in the body. It is also very important for growth in children and during pregnancy, and for mothers who are breast feeding. When treated appropriately those minor symptoms (like hair falling and soft fingernails) will also get better.

Magnesium, like Zinc, is also involved in a lot of metabolic functions (about 300 functions). Besides its role in regulating the blood sugar level, two other functions are very relevant and symptoms arising from deficiency are very common in the patients that I see. Firstly, when the Magnesium level is low, the patient gets very tired with very low energy. This is because Magnesium is needed in the metabolic cycle to produce energy. Even if the patients do not complain of poor energy levels they find that they have to struggle more to do the same thing that they used to do easily in the past, or they now need a longer rest period to recover. Secondly, the body (the muscles) cannot relax well when the Magnesium level is low. Patients often complain of feeling tense, anxious and not able to relax properly. They also have muscle aches, tension or cramps, and may have difficulty in falling asleep or staying asleep. Panic attacks have also been helped. Magnesium is important in heart muscle function and when low may result in abnormal rythms of the heart. It is also relevant, together with Calcium, in osteoporosis (thinning of the bones). I personally feel that if you are low in Magnesium it can make you more 'sensitive' as your body as a whole is more irritable. I also had patients complaining of tingling or other abnormal sensations on the skin such as super sensitivity to touch on the skin. Magnesium can also help you to stay calm. Thus you can see the importance of getting your Magnesium levels corrected when you are deficient in that mineral.

For some reasons, Zinc and Magnesium are used up more rapidly in our bodies than other nutrients, faster than can be supplied by the foods that are eaten. Among the patients I have seen over the years, a large proportion of them are low in these two nutrients, especially in older people.

Various tests can confirm the levels of these nutrients (such as testing the levels in blood or sweat), though with certain minerals the levels are reflected more accurately in certain fluids. For example with Magnesium, it is better to do a red cell Magnesium level test than just the serum level. With Zinc the sweat level is a better indicator than the serum level. Doing the serum levels alone does not accurately reflect the true status of these two minerals, for these tests emphasise overdose levels encountered in industrial poisoning.

Those who are on the contraceptive pill are at special risk of having low Zinc and Magnesium, as the pill is known to lower both these minerals in the body. They may also have other nutrient deficiencies but it is not in the remit of this book to talk about or cover them. If patients have symptoms relating to other nutrient deficiencies then I look into them specifically.

2) REESTABLISHING THE BALANCE OF MICROORGANISMS IN THE GUT

Probiotics

These are live microorganisms which when introduced into the gut would confer benefit and promote the balance of the live microorganisms in the gut—this is the scientific definition of a probiotic. On the practical level they are to help the gut function more efficiently. It is reckoned that there are more than 350 different species of the 'good' bacteria in the gut and they all perform different beneficial functions for the body. Scientists have only managed to isolate a proportion of them so far. The world was first alerted to the lactic acid bacteria by the Russian scientist Professor Metchnikoff in the early 20th.Century. He observed that certain people, especially those living in the Russian Steppes and in parts of Bulgaria, lived to a healthy old age. He postulated that there was a close connection with the sour milk that was part of the diet in those people. The bacteria that was subsequently isolated is called Lactobacillus Bulgaricus. Sour milk was very commonly prescribed for all kinds of tummy and other medical problems at one stage before the advent of antibiotics. Lactic acid bacteria seemed to alleviate these conditions, as the acid produced suppressed the invading bacteria. Sour milk was also regarded as an elixir for longevity (it was later shown not to be so) and Metchnikoff took it regularly, as did some of his friends.

Since then many other strains of bacteria have been isolated and shown to be beneficial in several medical conditions. Researches are still ongoing to firmly establish the claims made by the probiotics manufacturers for their products and to prove how different strains can help in different medical conditions. It is interesting to note that the food regulatory bodies in both Europe and USA have not accepted the medical claims made by the researchers on those products. The ECFS and FDA (the regulatory bodies) said that the evidence presented to them were insufficient for them to fully justify the claims. Therefore the labels can only state that the products may help in alleviating the stated medical conditions and cannot promise to be a cure for those conditions.

It is very important to take probiotics in the correct manner. There are many different manufacturers of probiotics, some have more strains of bacteria in their products, some less. They all are freeze-dried which means you have to give time to rehydrate them and reactivate them. In other words, after mixing the powder in water and stirring it, you must leave time for the bacteria to be reactivated. Otherwise they don't give the best intended result.

At this point it is appropriate for me to talk about the often asked question—what is the difference between probiotics and prebiotics? The answer in short: probiotics are living micro-organisms and prebiotics are the foods those micro-organisms need.

Prebiotics are non-digestible carbohydrate fibres that act as food for the probiotics. They stimulate and enhance the growth and activities of the intestinal bacteria to the benefit of the host. Two types of fibres are well recognised: the oligosaccharide and inulin. Both are fructo-oligosaccharides. Galactooligosaccharide, Mannan Oligosaccharide and Lactulose are also accepted as prebiotics. The following foods naturally contain prebiotics and probiotics. This is just for information and it is not mandatory that you should eat them unless you happen to like them.

Prebiotic foods
1) Most vegetables have inulin, those that have a higher amount (prebiotics) include :
    a) garlic
    b) onion
    c) leek
    d) artichoke
    e) chicory
    f) soya
2) Grains – which contain a high fibre content
    a) wheat
    b) barley
    c) oats

Probiotic foods
1) 'live' yoghurt
2) kefir - a blend of goat's milk and fermenting grains
3) sauerkraut - usually pickled cabbage
4) miso soup - a Japanese yeasty soup of fermented grains
5) tempeh - fermented soya
6) kimchi - Korean pickled vegetable
7) komboucha tea - Russian fermented drink

I remember that when I first started dealing with the Candida problem the only probiotic available widely was

Lactobaccilus Acidophilus but now the probiotic products in the market contain many strains. I would prefer a multi-strain product as the different species perform different beneficial functions and research has demonstrated their benefits in different medical conditions. Probiotics come in different forms: powder, capsules and tablets. I use the powder form as I think it is more effective The process used in turning living organisms into tablets must in my view affect the viability and efficacy of the bacteria in the tablet form and therefore I personally find tablets less preferable.

With the powder, you simply dissolve the powder in fluid, either water or milk. Water is the best fluid to rehydrate and re-activate the freeze-dried bacteria. After stirring the powder, leave it for a few minutes for the bacteria to become active again and drink it on a relatively empty stomach such as before breakfast or last thing at night. How often you need to take it would depend on the recommendation of the manufacturer of the different probiotics. Some probiotics are sold in capsule form to protect the bacteria from being destroyed by the hydrochloric acid during the passage through the stomach to the intestine. I doubt if the stomach acid destroys much of the bacteria because the loose powder (without encapsulation) has been used effectively to treat diarrhoea in children for many years, and also the bacteria themselves produce acid and can tolerate an acidic environment well.

For children (who have not learned to swallow tablets yet) I would have to use the probiotics powder. In the past I have used Nystatin (which has no side effects and with which I have never encountered any problems) in the liquid form for these patients. But because it is a proprietary drug some parents do not like it, and besides I think probiotics are a more appropriate treatment for patients of this age group.

Please note that vaginal and oral thrush need to be treated with the appropriate antifungals. Proprietary drugs have been used very successfully for many years for the treatment of these conditions.

I have often been asked whether probiotic-containing yoghurts are good things to eat. My view is that if you like them and can tolerate them, by all means have them, but you must realise that they are foods and not 'medicine'. If there is a medical problem it must be treated medically. The yoghurts may help to maintain a healthy gut simply because they are probiotic foods as stated above.

Other factors may also need to be considered. A change of lifestyle or steps taken to reduce stress (when that is identified as a triggering factor) are also very important. This is not necessary in the vast majority of patient, like those whose Candida imbalance was triggered by antibiotics or an incident of gastroenteritis (gut infection).

One common question that I am constantly asked is about the effect of antibiotics. Antibiotics are very important to combat infections. In very serious infections which are life threatening, you need them to save your life. The Candida problem which follows subsequently can be easily sorted out at a later stage. I obviously do not recommend the use of antibiotics for every minor ailment. If antibiotics are needed, it is useful to take an antifungal or probiotics alongside it or shortly after.

An Uncommon Species of Candida causing a problem

Caroline aged 27 came to me with a history of tummy bloating for the last 7 years. She had loose stools and low energy. She had been seen by a gastroenterologist and ultrasound of the abdomen together with endoscopies (examination of the gut with a flexible tube which has a camera attached) were carried out. These were all normal. With the usual treatment for the Candida problem her bowel movements became better and her energy improved. Her tummy bloating, though better, was still present and persisted. After a period of two months I sent her stools for a comprehensive analysis. I was glad when the results came back that she had a bacteria in the gut called Klebsiella pneumonia which can also ferment. This was duly treated with an antibiotic (Ciproxin) which the bacteria was sensitive to from the test of the stools. This helped initially but the bloating recurred after a while. A second course of antibiotics also did not prevent the abdominal bloating from recurring after a while. She did look 7 months pregnant from the bloating. A closer look at the stool test results showed a 1+ to Candida Inconspicua and Candida Ciferrii. The range is from 0 to 4+ (very significant infection). Normally a 1+ result, especially when it is stated non-pathogenic, can be ignored. In Caroline's case because the bloating was still recurrent, I thought that it might be worthwhile reviewing the stools result. I have not come across those species of Candida before but I thought it worth the while treating it. Those Candida species tested sensitive to 3 drug antifungals (Fluconazole, Itraconazole and Ketoconazole). I started her on a course of Fluconazole which is the safest of the 3, but this did not produce the desired result. I then used Itraconazole, and after a few days on it, for the first time in years her bloating disappeared and her abdomen was flat as it should be for a young lady. This showed that occasionally some unexpected species of Candida may interfere with the expectation of a good response when treating the Candida imbalance, and the right antifungal then needs to be used to combat the outstanding Candida species.

Once the Candida problem comes under control it does not mean it will not flare up again, because the many triggering factors are beyond our control. However, next time it gets into a state of imbalance you will know what to do, having been through the treatment regime previously. You will recognise the symptoms earlier and be able to take the necessary remedial steps and make the changes in your life much more quickly than before. A short course of Caprilic Plus would also be very helpful to get the situation under control once again. I also advise patients to take the Caprilic Plus whenever they have had too much of the wrong foods, or when they are away on holiday and do not want to be too careful with what they eat, or when they are invited to dinner and do not know what they will be served.

7

CANDIDA AND CHILDREN

CHILDREN WITH THE PROBLEM

Children are also susceptible to the Candida problem. In conventional medicine children are not viewed as mini-adults with disease. There are medical conditions that only affect children and not adults and vice-versa. With regard to the Candida problem they are just mini-adults except that they do not usually have multiple symptoms and fewer triggering factors, as they are still young. The most common triggering factor is antibiotics which give rise to tummy upsets. The most common medical complaints are those related to the gastrointestinal tract and the skin. As they grow older they may develop symptoms like in the adults.

Jimmy's mother's story
She wrote:
    As promised, a brief note about Jimmy—his condition etc when we came to see you and now.

Before Dr.Choy
We first came to see you in September 2010. Jimmy had

been diagnosed with Eosinophilic Oesophagitis and Gastro-Oesophageal Reflux when he was 3 years old (2006) from an endoscopy and ph studies. After a short course of Omeprazole, things seemed to settle down only for it to recur in 2008, when again he was given another short course of Omeprazole. Ultimately, aged 7 years (2010), his episodes of reflux had become so severe and his willingness to eat reducing, that we returned to the specialist for another endoscpy in July 2010. The reflux index was 4.4 to 11.1 percent on different days. We were referred to a dietician who suggested eliminating the following foods from his (already severly reduced diet): wheat, dairy, soya, gluten, shellfish and sugar. I refused on the ground that it was impossible to do and would cause further mental hang-ups overeating. We were then advised to take a longer course of Omeprazole and to swallow a nebule of 250 mcg viscous Budesonide daily. Again I refused this course of action based on his age and the potential side effects.

At this point, September 2010, Jimmy's reflux meant he had to visit the loo to spit out what was in his mouth, usually about one teaspoon full. This happened during meals, whilst playing sports and often at nights and other times of the day. He complained of nausea and tummy pain and was increasingly reluctant to eat, especially foods he was unfamiliar with. He also itched a lot and had large grey circles under his eyes.

After Dr.Choy

You gave him probiotics daily and reduced his dairy intake. In February 2011 we sought the help of K.M. In helping him to gain confidence in eating. She diagnosed a food phobia as a result of the pain caused by the OE and Gastric Reflux. She spent four days with Jimmy, cooking, talking about food and trying new foods. Gradually Jimmy began to trust more food types. This would never have been possible had his condition not improved significantly under your care.

Now, June 2012, he takes probiotics daily. He has not had any reflux (reaching his throat and therefore aware of it) for almost a year. He has grown in confidence and now eats much more, albeit less than most children. He does occasionally have a bout of regurgitation but this is often because he rushes his food and doesn't chew properly—a small boy wanting to go back outside and play football.

Because of his remarkable progress he had been able to start full boarding school, something we didn't think possible because of his severe reluctance to eat. The probiotics are easily administered by the school nurse/matron and he takes a full part in all areas of school life.

We are really indebted to you for all you have done for Jimmy. We were in a bad place when we first came to see you and I really didn't know where to turn. My only regret is not having found you when he was first diagnosed aged 3.

Jimmy's mother

The above story shows that children also suffer from the effects of the Candida problem. Unlike adults the majority of children that I have seen presented with symptoms of the gastrointestinal system. Babies can get oral thrush and infants do get nappy rash. Occasionally they present with skin complaint (eczema) or other symptoms.

Tummy pains
This is a very common complaint with the children that I have seen. Often the tummy ache comes on after breakfast

before going to school. This naturally leads to parents wondering whether the children do not want to go to school and are therefore making up the symptoms, or they have something real to account for the symptoms. Whilst there may be other minor incidental factors, the gas resulting from Candida fermentation can stretch the small intestine and cause acute colicky pain. The problem will subside when treated.

Selina was aged 12 when her mother brought her to see me because of persistent tummy pains. From the age of 2 she had eczema and asthma and these symptoms were managed with conventional medication. It was not till her menarche (first menstrual period) at age 9, that everything was exacerbated. Besides her eczema and asthma getting worse, she also developed tummy pains with diarrhoea and headache and tiredness. She was given a total of 10 courses of antibiotics to no avail and was eventually referred to a private paediatrician (child specialist). Here her mother had to spend lots of money on various tests and was eventually told that everything was fine—except that blood tests showed that Selina was allergic to many foods. The only way to get her better was to avoid those many foods. This course of action made her feel miserable as she could not join her friends during lunch time and had to eat different foods separately. This did not lead her to feeling better and she was eventually recommended to see me. I sorted out her Candida problem and within 4 months I was asked to write a letter to her school stating that she was now able to join the other pupils at lunch and eat normally, except for a reduced sugar and yeast intake. She continues to eat normally with no recurrence of symptoms and has remained well since.

I saw *Henry*, aged 2, with his parents a few years ago. He had been having loose stools and frequent diarrhoea and the occasional tummy ache since he was 6 months old. His parents brought him to see a paediatric gastroenterologist and lots of investigations were carried out costing a lot of money. All investigations came back negative and he was put on a diet avoiding wheat, eggs and dairy products. That did not seemed to have made much difference to his condition and his loose bowel movements persisted. I treated him for Candida and prescribed probiotics and within a very short while, improvements were noticed. When I saw him again 4 weeks later, his father was pleased to be able to say that Henry's stools were no longer loose and he had not mentioned a single time that his tummy hurt him. His father initially brought him to see me on the recommendation of a family friend whose son was also of a similar age with similar complaints. He had also spent a great deal of money on investigations which were negative and did not help with his son's symptoms. When he was treated for the Candida overgrowth his symptoms resolved.

The lesson that came out of these cases showed that for those who are financially restricted, a different route can be taken first. Investigations are relevant and I fully support them. Even though they may not tell you what is causing the problem, at least you know what is not causing the problem when the tests are negative. My view is that if the child has recurrent tummy symptoms he should be seen by a doctor first, to rule out any acute surgical condition. If it is deemed not to be acute, the child can be given probiotics regularly and told to cut out sugar as best as possible. (I have never put children on diet for the Candida problem except to avoid sugar as best as possible). In children the response is usually quite quick. If after two weeks nothing seems to change then further investigations will be necessary to get to the bottom of the problem. In this way you would spare the child the ordeal of tests which can be disturbing especially to younger children, not to mention the financial cost involved.

Constipation

By the time I see these children they have usually been on laxatives for some time to treat the problem of constipation without much result. In some children this started to happen after they had come out of nappies; this make some parents wonder whether there is some correlation with poor potty training. Whatever the reason is, treating the Candida did seem to solve the problem in those children I have seen.

Mrs. T brought her daughter who was then aged 4 to see me. She (the child) had been suffering from constipation for the past 2 years and had been seen by the paediatrician. Various medications were prescribed over a period of time but they did not have much effect on the problem. I thought she had a Candida problem and gave her Candida neutralising drops and probiotics. When I saw her again a month later, her bowels were working fine and regular at once a day.

16 months later Mrs. T came with her son who was nearly aged 4 who also had problems with constipation but only for the last few months. Again the Candida problem was treated and the constipation was resolved.

3 weeks later she came with another daughter aged 9 who also had constipation for the last few months. The problem abated once again when the Candida problem was sorted out.

Mrs.T has 2 other younger children who had not

complained yet of constipation, but I recommended that they take probiotics regularly for a couple of months to keep the gut balanced.

Nausea and not wanting to eat
I put these two symptoms together because they are linked in the cases I have seen. Excess Candida increases the amount of gas from the fermentation which can fill up the stomach causing a pressure difference between the stomach and the outside of the body. Throwing up is the only way to equalise the pressure difference to relieve the symptom thus making the patients feel nauseous and being sick. If the stomach is filled with gas, you feel full and cannot eat and you are therefore reluctant to eat.

Aaron, aged nearly 3 when I saw him, was born 5 weeks prematurely. To keep him alive doctors had to give him various medications including antibiotics for other life threatening medical conditions. His main symptoms when I saw him were nausea and not eating. When his Candida problem was sorted out, the nausea disappeared and he was eating and putting on weight once again, making his parents very happy again.

Sugar craving
Kevin aged 9 came to see me with his mother. The main complaint being weight gain and a strong craving for sugar over the last few months. His mother also noticed that Kevin tended to stutter after he had sugar. His other symptoms were an eczematous rash on the skin and scabby scalp. He was treated in the same way as with other children with the Candida problem.

When I saw them again a few months later, his mother said that Kevin was able to keep away from sugar and his sugar craving was gone. His weight had been steady, and his skin and scalp were much better. His mother was very pleased with his improvement and then revealed that Kevin had been doing badly at school previously. Recently his teacher had remarked that something had changed in Kevin, his concentration had improved tremendously and his class performance had been very much better. He does not stutter now except when he has had too much sugar. This part of his symptoms was not made known at the original consultation as his mother thought that Kevin's class performance was just the way Kevin was and she was too ashamed to tell anybody that. Anyway Kevin remains well and continues to do well in class.

Other symptoms such as in adults are far less common but they do happen in children. I have seen many children who developed the Candida problem after a rapid growth spurt. The triggering factors in most other cases are about the same as in adults though the history of antibiotics intake is the most common reason. Next is a history of tummy upset whether due to food poisoning or gastroenteritis caused by bacteria or virus.

I have never put a child on a diet except to ask the parents to restrict the sugar intake of the child as best as they can. It is clear that in most cases the Candida imbalance did not happen because they ate badly, but once there is Candida overgrowth then sugars make their problems worse. Putting them on Probiotics will usually resolve the symptoms they have. Caprilic Plus is not suitable for these younger people as they cannot swallow the capsules. Probiotics come in the powder form and are mixed in water, so there is no capsules to swallow.

86

8

NEUTRALISATION TREATMENT

A SIMPLE AND EFFECTIVE WAY OF TREATMENT

Patients are given high dilution extracts of Candida—to be taken 0.05ml orally two or three times a day depending on the severity of their symptoms. This is not always necessary as part of their treatment. I have many patients who live abroad, and as I cannot monitor them closely I do not give them these drops, or I give them drops for just the first month. However they respond just as well with the rest of the treatment. These drops, or 'vaccines', are of homeopathic dilutions and are very safe. This is not homeopathic treatment but is more like immunisation. I liken it to homeopathy only in that the solution used is of a great dilution. The treatment dose or 'end point' dose may need to be adjusted depending on how well the patient responds and that is why I do not give drops, or only one course of drops to overseas patients, as I am unable to see them regularly to adjust the dosage. I have found that those who are on these drops seem to respond a little bit faster compared to those without 'drops' but they all respond in the end.

The principle of this 'vaccines' is based on the intradermal (injections into the skin) technique of provocation—neutralisation as improved by Dr. Joseph Miller some fifty years ago and used by doctors successfully in treating allergies in several parts of the world. When I first started using this technique, and had personally done hundreds of these tests (injections), that allowed me to observe patients closely, their reactions and responses, and my assessment on this technique. I also had the opportunity to meet Dr. Miller and spend a couple of days at Dr. Miller's clinic at Alabama, USA, discussing with him the technique, and observing him at work and the results he gets with this technique. That was nearly 36 years ago.

I adapted his technique to one without using injections thirty-two years ago, using the muscle testing technique. With the Miller method, a small amount of the suspected antigen (0.05ml) is injected under the skin (intradermally) and the resultant wheal noted: hard, soft or flat. If the patient is affected by the antigen (food or chemical), symptoms can be provoked and the resultant wheal on the skin will be hard. Higher serial dilutions of that antigen are then subsequently injected until the provoked symptoms are neutralised and the resulting wheal becomes soft, not flat.This is then the neutralising or treatment dose, and the treatment is injecting 0.05 ml of the prepared solution—allergy shots as the Americans call them—subcutaneously (deeper under the skin) once or twice a day depending on the medical indications.

These testings and treatment (injections) can be a highly unpleasant experience and very time-consuming and labour intensive, and therefore can be expensive. Using the muscle testing technique I can arrive at the same point in a fraction of the time needed (compared to the standard method) and without provoking any symptom. I have used this method for thirty- two years now and my observation is that the 'end point' reached is much more appropriate and suitable to the patients. This is also non-invasive and a patient-friendly method, and children don't run away as they did with the injections. As far as I know nobody does this in exactly the same way as I do (I have done it this way for the past 32 years). There are many doctors who do the intradermal testing all over the world.

Patients take these drops orally, usually for a couple of months and when they are better, the frequency of taking the drops can be reduced and then stopped when their symptoms have all resolved.

9

LETTERS FROM PATIENTS

GRATEFUL PATIENTS RELATING THEIR EXPERIENCES

I have included several letters from patients to illustrate the link between the Candida problem and seemingly unrelated symptoms. The letters are reproduced exactly as they have been written by the patients. They have not been altered in any way except the names have been changed. These letters were written by grateful former patients who want to tell others what they have been through and how sorting out the Candida problem changed their lives.

Letter number one

Danny, aged 45, had complaints of not feeling right for the last few years. He had a persistent 'hangover' and so he hardly drank alcohol, his brain didn't work well and his concentration was very bad. He was treated and below is his letter:

Danny's letter

Just a short note to thank you for the Candida treatment you have provided me. I am feeling clear minded, and more able to cope with the stresses and pressures of work and everyday life. My sleep patterns and my general wellbeing is better than it has been for many many years.

Being mainly a believer in traditional medicine, I have to say I was extremely skeptical to begin with. My wife suggested I come to see you after having cured her allergy to our newly acquired pet dog. I found you straight talking and your no nonsense approach very welcoming.

Danny

Letter number two

Penny lives in Ireland and her letter talks about her skin symptoms and what she went through.

Penny's letter

Thank you so much for your help and advice. My problem started 3 years ago with large painful blisters on the sole of my right foot and then a couple of days later on the palms of both hands. I couldn't walk properly and open my hands properly as the blisters were so painful.

My GP lanced the blisters to provide some relief and referred me to a skin specialist in Dublin who did blood tests and took a biopsy of the skin and also a sample of the fluid for analysis. Later when I saw him again, he said he couldn't make a definitive diagnosis as all the test results were negative. He suggested it might be an auto-immune reaction and prescribed steroids. He advised that I reduced the steroids after 3 weeks. The steroids worked but the blisters came back every time I tried to reduce the dose. I couldn't afford to take steroids long term as we have a strong family history of osteoporosis and I have been told that long term steroids affect bone density.

I came to see you in London on the recommendation of

my sister in law. You advised a diet avoiding sugar and to take the antifungal (Caprilic Plus). You also advised me to reduce the steroid gradually. My GP was very sceptical but within 3 months I was able to stop the steroids completely without a flare up of the skin condition. There has not been a recurrence of the problem since.

Now when I get pain and tingling which are early symptoms of the skin condition, I take a short course of Caprilic Plus and reduce sugar in my diet and the blisters don't happen.

Penny

I just want to let people know that a simple problem such as the Candida overgrowth can lead to a baffling skin condition but more importantly it can be treated easily.

Letter number three

Zara's symptoms are not too uncommon but not every sufferer has the Candida problem.

Zara's letter

I contracted a virus aged 17 that initially had flu like symptoms and a fever. I thought I would get better within a couple of weeks. Eight weeks after the illness started I was still in bed and could hardly walk down the stairs. Conventional GPs did not know why I was still ill and diagnosed ME/chronic fatigue but did not know of a way to treat it.

Having seen multiple different medical and other practitioners I eventually came to Dr. Choy about 18 months after developing the original virus. At this point I was functioning and able to walk and had done my A levels but was still extremely ill. He diagnosed both a severe Candida problem and a Magnesium deficiency. One of the worst symptoms I had experienced was an inability to concentrate and a tendency to get bad headaches if I read for more than half an hour. I also had problems remembering what was at the beginning of a paragraph by the time I had got to the end of it. Dr. Choy put this down to the Candida problem and prescribe Caprilic Plus to sort it out. The effect of taking the Caprilic Plus is very unpleasant and they are very strong and make you feel sick. However they did sort out the problem and gradually the symptoms decreased. This undoubtedly helped my immune system recover over the long term. In the short term my reliance on Magnesium tablets was very great and for a couple of years I had to take 10-14 tablets every day. This had now decreased and I only need to take them when my system is down. (Author's comment—please note that Zara was taking food state Magnesium which is different from other types of Magnesium). The Candida problem has not returned after the original was sorted out.

I am really sorry for my woefully slow response in all respects of your request. My only excuse is that your treatment resulted in my full recovery to the point that I now work in an investment bank where you work very long hours and it somewhat takes over your life.

I love my job and I am extremely grateful for all the help you gave. Kind regards,

Zara

Letter number four

Lorraine is a retired GP who had been in the front line dealing with patients at the general practitioner level for forty years. In her letter she relates her symptoms and her response to the Candida treatment.

Lorraine's letter

I am most grateful to you for your kindness and treatment of me when I was at a very low ebb.

I have Addison's disease (which affects the adrenal glands) diagnosed 30 years ago, and have taken several courses of antibiotics for chest infections. I also have osteoporosis as a side effect of steroid replacement therapy.

About 4 years ago I started to experience bowel symptoms with attacks of abdominal discomfort, often severe colic, followed by increasing bowel looseness and frequently diarrhoea. This was accompanied by nausea and anorexia. The episodes would last for 24 to 48 hours and would occur every week or so. Between bouts my stomach always felt uncertain. I became increasingly unsure about going out and was unhappy if I couldn't sit on the end of a row in the theatre etc... I remember a trip to Venice 2 years ago when I swear I knew the location of every loo. I lost weight and had little energy or appetite.

Eventually in October 2010 I saw a gastroenterologist, had a colonoscopy (a camera to look at the large intestine) and irritable bowel was diagnosed. I tried various over the counter remedies and various diets. A gluten free diet helped in the short term and a dairy free (as opposed to lacto free) diet certainly helped.

Finally in desperation and thinking I was burdened with this for the rest of my life I came to see you. You said that you thought this was Candida and gave Caprillic Plus which I took in July 2011. It made things worse for a time but about a fortnight after finishing the medication most of the symptoms disappeared. You then gave me Probiotics which caused a slight relapse but after finishing them I again became and have remained symptom free apart from very mild episodes if I eat excess amount of sugar or dairy products. I find the difference in my life unbelievable, and apart from avoiding dairy products suffer no inconvenience.

I am and shall remain ever grateful.

Kindest regards,

Lorraine

Letter number five

Frederica is a 28 year old American graduate in laboratory science who came over to the UK on a work contract. Here is her interesting story.

Frederica's letter

My symptoms began on the evening of 26th December 2011. I developed a rash on my right shoulder. The rash was slightly raised and it had a burning sensation. I called the NHS helpline and they thought I was having an allergic reaction and I was advised to take some Benadryl. By the following morning the rash was gone. About two weeks later I developed a bump on my spine. Again I took some Benadryl and the bump was gone although the area was still a little red the following morning but I soon put it out of my mind. But by the end of January I began to have swollen joints for a day or two. At first I thought it was an injury but then it became more frequent and I made an appointment with my GP. I saw my GP on the 27th February. He thought the rash was due to an allergic reaction and prescribed an antihistamine (Loratadine 10mg) although he was unsure of what caused the joint swelling and pain. At that point he thought the urticaria and swelling may be unrelated.

After being on the antihistamine for several days, I knew that it wasn't working and my symptoms became worse. I went back to my GP and he ordered some blood tests. Two days later, I went back to my GP, this time both my knees were swollen and it was difficult to walk. He was finally able to see the swelling for the first time and thought I had Erythema Nodosum. He prescribed me 15mg of Prednisolone twice a day for 10 days. This appeared to make the swelling stop although I still had some urticaria that week. Once I finished the 10 days course of medication, my symptoms came back even worse than before. I was put on a different antihistamine (Fexofenadine 120mg) and more blood tests were ordered but again everything came back normal. I then asked to be referred to an allergy specialist. By now I was having symptoms every day and I had to call in sick a few times because the swelling made it difficult to walk or even hold a pen. I also began to develop new symptoms that felt as if my legs were on fire. Also, my energy levels were really low and I had lost more than a stone in weight.

I was finally referred to Professor C and decided to keep a food diary until my appointment on the 10th of April. Based on my food diary, Professor C suggested avoiding wheat and dairy. After avoiding the foods for a few days, I felt much better. By the time I saw Professor C again on the 1st of May, I felt even better although the list of foods I had to avoid was fairly large.

I was also referred to Professor H (a skin specialist with particular experience in urticaria) for more testing, but those tests came back normal. He did suggest increasing my dose of Fexofenadine to 180mg twice a day, since I still had some occasional urticaria. The list of foods to avoid was very long and it kept growing. I also began to have daily urticaria again and noticed I was very gassy. I began to wonder if this was really food allergies and knew something was really wrong after I felt unwell after just having a little white rice and some water. I saw Professor C again on the 31st of May and he referred me to Dr. Choy.

I saw Dr. Choy on the 1st June and he said my problems could be due to Candida overgrowth. Although I am unsure as to what may have triggered the Candida problem—it may have started after a bout of severe food poisoning I had in India in May 2010. Dr. Choy tested my Candida level and found that it was too high to treat in the usual way. So I began to take probiotics, zinc, magnesium and changed my diet. I had to avoid all foods that caused the urticaria and also avoid sugar. I decided to avoid carbs as much as possible since he felt this may help. After two weeks, my Candida level had dropped low enough to be treated with Caprilic Plus. I began to eat carbs again and I slowly began to introduce the foods that gave me reactions before. By the 22nd July I was no longer taking Fexofenadine. I still had occasional urticaria , but it was much more mild than before and I felt much better. By the end of August, I was able to eat gluten again. Unfortunately I thought I was healed and had some sugar too early, causing my symptoms to come back. However, the Candida level appears to be decreasing again and I am sure I will be healed soon.

Last September I moved back to the United States after my work contract in the UK ended. Since moving back I have noticed that both my aunt and her granddaughter have developed urticaria and swelling within the past year and have been diagnosed as having food allergies. Although my aunt is on antihistamines, she still has urticaria. She has never had any food allergies before this year. Her granddaughter is only 10 years old, so she may have developed food allergies, but I wonder if they have a Candida problem instead of food allergies like I did.

Yours sincerely,
Frederica

Letter number six

Susie recalls the frustration at not being able to get the appropriate advice and treatment for her symptoms.

Susie's letter

The symptoms that I had for years were that of a hugely bloating stomach which I could never pinpoint why and what foods caused it as I was keeping off acidic foods, pasta, gluten etc. etc. Having seen various gastro consultants and a nutritionist over time and been told that I was either fat or had IBS, no one ever suggested it could be Candida and as you are aware, you totally saved the day and cutting yeast and sugar out of my diet reformed life completely for me. I used to go into endless good health food shops trying to eat the correct foods and closely followed the Ayurveda diet from Dr. J's book at one stage, but no avail. I had previously purchased a really good juicer to try and just have pure good fruit and vegetable smoothies, but nothing worked.

I just became more and more exasperated and frustrated that I was throwing so much hard-earned money away on absolutely nothing and still having awful stomach pain and huge bloating. I also had regular visits to have colonics which never really helped, until one time when I was in total agony and had an urgent appointment and felt less sore after, but not for long.

The Candida diet was a hugely strict regime as yeast and sugar are in so many items that we eat in daily life. Initially it was hard but I stuck to it rigidly and the results were quick to show. For the first time in YEARS I started to feel better without the painful stomach ache, lack of energy, stomach never really working and actually losing weight. Despite undertaking exercise on a daily basis, I always had this protruding stomach and could never lose weight. Not only is my stomach very bloated but at times would just blow up like a balloon and I could easily look 6 months pregnant, but also in my face.

When we were on holidays in Portugal, a few months prior to seeing you, I was drinking quite a bit of white wine and my feet just blew up and were hugely itchy and blotchy with patches of where I had scratched, and painful too which would keep me awake at night. Although I purchased some antifungal crea, nothing really helped, but I believe from our conversations that that was due to the Candida toxins affecting the feet. Fortunately I have never suffered from vaginal thrush. Having seen you recently, you advised that due to my hormones the Candida was coming back slightly, and interestingly I have noticed that my toes and feet are again swelling now and again with the blotching, itching and redness.

As I have mentioned to you previously, there were numerous advices (which tended to be American), but no definite list of what I could and could not eat when I first saw you, but managed to find one list on the Internet of foods to eat and foods to avoid that was very strict and I decided to follow this as my main base and kept to it as the most helpful and logical. There was no book that really helped either, hence I think this book will be so helpful to sufferers.

Also, quite early on after seeing you, I started to take Kefir (the fermented milk). Initially I took a good glass or two of this in one day and was violently ill for the next 24 hours, but I felt it removed a lot of rubbish from my stomach and then subsequently had a glass of it every morning which I found helped my stomach movements hugely. I stopped when I went through my IVF treatment and early pregnancy but at 7 months pregnant have started to have a small amount again along with your probiotic powder. I did wonder if the state of my stomach with a huge build up of Candida (which I did not realise at the time), was something that added to a cause when I had a miscarriage.

Having struggled so much to lose weight over the years and trying to feel better, from starting your diet on 22nd December and finishing it in March prior to IVF treatment, I lost 20lbs over that time, which was a miracle for me. To feel so much better was amazing.

Kind regards,

Susie

Letter number seven

Veronica was aged 28 when I first saw her. She had a whole range of health issues from facial acne to headaches and was desperate to have children. When the Candida was sorted out, all her symptoms subsided and her skin was cleared of acne and became smooth again. Below is what she wants to say.

Veronica's letter

Nine years ago when I met Dr. Choy I did not realise how much my health would improve. I am now the happy mother of three beautiful healthy children who rarely need to go and see a doctor. As a child I had asthma which needed inhalers and antibiotics. In my teens I developed quite bad acne and had severe period pains. Then in my early twenties I developed irritable bowel syndrome, polycystic ovarian syndrome and anxiety issues. When I look back now I realise how much my diet had an effect on my health and my perception that the doctor had all the answers.

At my first appointment with Dr. Choy I was suffering from polycystic ovarian syndrome (POC), Irritable bowel syndrome (IBS)and fertility problems. We had been married nine months and very eager to start a family. I had kept track of my menstrual cycle every month but soon realised this could vary from 27 to 37 days. The 37 day cycle was the worse as each time you think maybe this month is the one. But when it was not the feeling was tough which led to craving even more chocolate and sweet foods which only made the IBS worse. In the middle of this you were trying to work and keep a happy face so no one knew how you felt. The sugar cravings then led to extreme tiredness especially mid-afternoon and when the tiredness hit in the only way I thought I could fight it was eating more sugar laden food. This kept me going until around 6 o'clock when I got home from work and crashed onto the sofa and could easily fall asleep for an hour. I rarely woke up in the morning feeling full of energy for the day ahead.

When we went out with friends I found I was reacting more and more to alcohol. I could get very drunk easily which could lead onto vomiting or falling asleep. The after effects could start an episode of IBS which could last days and I was going around in a fog.. I now know that this was my body trying to deal with Candida and unresolved emotional issues.

The POC developed gradually over the years from period pains to to acne to hormonal sweats then lumps in my breast which had to be removed. When I asked a GP for help with POC I was told I could go back on a different contraceptive pill even though I had just said I was trying to get pregnant

I was nervous but willing to listen and try anything when Dr. Choy first started testing with my arm. I had not heard of Candida before but when I listened to the symptoms of fluctuating blood sugar levels and cravings for sugar it all started to make sense. I was told to cut out wine, beer, bananas, grapes, melons honey & dried fruit. Initially I thought it would be hard but with the help of the drops, zinc, magnesium, caprylic acid & chromium I began to feel more energetic and healthy.

The next nine months were up and down as I saw Dr. Choy every four to six weeks and continued to have my Candida levels checked along with my vitamin levels. The POC and IBS did improve and my sugar cravings were greatly reduced. I had a lot more energy and I felt a cloud had been lifted from my head as well as I begun to see thinks more clearly. What I thought were big worries were actually put into perspective.

Eight months after my first appointment in a cold January day I was starting to doubt if this Candida programme was working. I had spent Christmas and New year avoiding alcohol and sugary foods and I was still not pregnant. Dr. Choy told me my candida levels were the lowest they had been and I had a good chance of getting pregnant in the following few months. The next month I got the news we had been waiting 18 months to hear—I was pregnant. I continued to see Dr. Choy thoughout the pregnancy taking two zinc, one for me and one for the baby and then an Essential fatty acid supplement for the last few months. I had a great pregnancy and a beautiful healthy baby girl at the end.

My Candida symptoms did come back after the baby was born but this time I knew the signals from my body and could address them with Dr. Choy's support. When I discussed the possibility of baby number 2 with my husband and I thought I was entering into another long haul of trying to get pregnant. This time first month and baby number two was on her way! Again I had a very healthy pregnancy with Dr. Choy monitoring my zinc & iron levels. When baby number two was born I thought her tummy was slightly bloated and she had a lot of wind even though she was being breastfed. At five weeks old when I was seeing Dr. Choy for myself I asked him to check her for Candida. She did have it but the probiotic powder helped her. I am now aware of this and know her Candida signals and will hopefully be able to support her so that she does not have to go through the same Candida battle that I had.

Baby number 3 also came 1 month after trying and I also had a very healthy pregnancy and baby. My husband and I will always be very grateful to the support, advice and help we got from Dr. Choy. It is such a shame that more doctors do not recognise the symptoms of Candida and the power Candida can have on your body when left untreated.

Veronica

Letter number eight

Vicky, whom I have referred to earlier, is of Eastern European origin and English is not her mother tongue. She is a geologist by profession and works for an international oil company. She is now 49 years of age and her mother was a practising doctor in her country. Her letter contains expressions which are not very English and grammatically incorrect and with some spelling mistakes. Nevertheless I have reproduced it word for word. She has a story to tell which is very interesting.

Vicky's letter

My allergy saga, once identified, lasted more than twelve years! During that time I lived in five different European countries where I have been looking for help at numerous allargologist (allergists). In that period a few allergies were confirmed but the long treatments (very time consuming) that were conducted were unsuccessful. The symptoms were very diverse, fluctuating by type and strength during the

103

years and not always being typical allergy symptoms. In addition I realised that some of the symptoms manifested at first when I have been six years old. My various pains brought me over the years to ortopedicians (orthopaedics surgeon), gastroenterologist, cardiologist, dermatologist, ophtalmologist (ophthalmologist), pulmonlogist (chest specialist). As they never managed to find the cause of my complains the only outcome was that I was considered hypochondriac and not taken seriously. Meanwhile I was living in constant pain and excessive tiredness for which (I) needed regularly 10 hours sleep a day. In my late twenties I developed the very real feeling that if I am loosing my strength due to ageing in that way I will not reach my 45th birthday. What is worse, that feeling didn't make me sad as my life was a struggle to survive any (every) single day which was making it pointless. My health problems affected my life in any (every) single day. Once it became clear that all the problems are somehow allergy related the search became more channeled. I was reacting to all foods apart from five types, to all air allergens, all the chemicals in the food and in the air so was diagnosed as polyallergic. (Still) I could not believe that I am allergic to everything and keep asking the question Why? What? How? I was convinced that something triggers it all.

When relocated to UK, was referred to Dr. Choy by another allergologist. Dr. Choy did not want to know all my diagnosis history, only my symptoms. I should admit that his diagnostic method was a bit unusual and raised my eyebrow. However Dr. Choy made me feel comfortable and I feel I can trust him. In addition his diagnosis coincided with the one some of the conventional allergologist defined. The treatment was the same, but with homeopathic medicaments (dilutions). The doctor determined that what is the main problem was the allergy to Candida Albican and suggested treating it first. So I decided to give it a try and it was rewiring. In five days my symptoms subsided considerably and in two weeks time I had a very active life. Ten months after the treatment initiated I climbed without any problem Uhuru peak of Kilimanjaro mountain, achievement that I never dreamed of.

In fourteen I was desensitised and my vaccine and medicaments were stopped. It took several more months to desensitise the other allergies and now after a bit more than two years I am no longer the sick person I was. I am like anyone else! Even in my most daring dream I didn't dream to feel so healthy. And how I could have? I didn't know that this is the way a healthy person should feel! I no longer feel half of my body in pain and I am not even aware that I have joints, bones and organs as the pain from them every single minute of the day in the past would remind me of their presence. Every day I thank Dr. Choy for making my life as wonderful as I never imagined life can be.

I should note (say) that I had undergone a conventional medicaments treatment (fungizone and subcutaneous vaccination) for three and a half years without any positive result. But Dr. Choy's homeopathic medicaments and personal (titrated for each individual) worked wonders.

And I was right: I was not allergy to everything! It was the Candida Albican that was making me feel miserable. So the suggestion I can give to all allergic people is: do not give up and (but) try any treatment. You do not know what will work. You can be healthy as well.

Vicky

Letter number nine

Alice has written outlining her experience during her bad times and how she gradually recovered. Her letter shows how the Candida problem can lead to all kinds of secondary adverse reactions to foods.

Alice's letter

It started after an evening out with friends. We'd eaten spicy oriental food at a London noodle bar and when I got home I felt short of breath. I thought perhaps it was asthma but I'd never had asthma before and didn't understand what was happening to me. In a bit of a panic I phoned the emergency NHS number and told them I was suffering an allergy attack. They told me to take antihistamines, which I did, and soon I could breathe normally again.

I remained terrified. I simply didn't know what I was eating that was causing the problem, and therefore how to stop the same thing happening again. I became wary of foods in general and almost stopped eating, with the result that I lost loads of weight.

My GP referred me to an allergy expert for testing, but agonisingly the appointment was months away. When I finally did see him—and he was one of the most eminent specialists in the UK—he told me I was allergic to more than 30 different foods, including avocados, tomatoes, bananas, melon, broccoli, all nuts (apart from peanuts, ironically) chestnuts, ginger, spices, shellfish, sugar, peppers and asparagus. These were but a few of the things I could no longer enjoy.

In addition, there were also environmental allergens; several medicines including antibiotics and aspirin, and drugs to treat hayfever, would send me into shock. I was also allergic to latex. The diagnosis was devastating. It appeared that there was nothing I could eat or touch, nowhere I could safely go. The world had turned on me and I couldn't imagine how I would manage. When I asked how serious my reactions would be to all these newly prohibited substances, the specialist said to avoid everything completely.

There was—although I didn't realise it at the time—a single flicker of hope. My specialist said in 'complicated' cases like mine that one should see Dr. Choy, an allergist he recommended only to his 'trickier' patients. By this time, I'd suffered a further incident of anaphylactic shock after eating a cake which I didn't realise contained traces of ginger. I was really at my wits end, terrified of eating anything anything and down to 7 stones in weight (I'm 5'5') and size 6-8 in clothes. I was already 2 stones below my normal weight. I couldn't understand what was going on with my body, or why, and I had the feeling of being helpless and at the mercy of these advancing allergies. It impacted my entire life.

Then, as soon as I met Dr. Choy, things started to come together. He muscle tested me (which at that time I found illogical) and told me to stay off all sugar producing foods and some fruits. He prescribed me an anti-fungal tablet, Nystatin, for some months and told me I had to change my life! Then he explained how I can do that. I suppose he may have also given me Zinc supplements at that time, but I can't precisely remember now. His approach was holistic in that he asked about my lifestyle, emotions and my medical history. I understood from him that I had displayed 'symptoms' for years and years without realising it. During that time I had somehow accumulated an excessive amount of Candida in my body, which had disturbed my immune system and was the cause of my allergic reactions and a bunch of other concurrent symptoms.

When I looked back with the benefit of this new information, I could see my allergic symptoms had actually started in my teens. I realised that since then I had often visited my GP complaining of a certain pain in the lower right hand side of my stomach—an occasional cramping and a constant dull pain. I always suspected a grumbling appendix but my concern was always dismissed: apparently I had no problem, but the pain felt real and it's cause remained unidentified. Gradually, it was suggested I was anxious—that it was all in my head. I felt I was dismissed as a hypochondriac. That was in the 1980s.

In my early twenties I 'suddenly' became allergic to cats (despite having lived with them since childhood) and experienced for the first time very bad hay fever, which seemed to increased annually in severity. For years, I took antihistamines every day of the summer and over the years they grew less and less effective. My diet as a young adult had been poor. I rarely cooked properly and mostly ate takeaways (Chinese or Indian). I swallowed chocolate and sweets religiously. I seemed to live on carbohydrates—bread and pasta with ketchup were favourites. But it was OK: I was thin, I had a fast metabolism, I was active and ate a lot. Food was fuel.

In 1992, at the age of 24, I moved to Eastern Europe where the food was 'local' and quite restricted in terms of vegetables and the breath of choice I'd been brought up with in the West. There were no Chinese or Indian dishes (those cuisines were unavailable so soon after the iron curtain had been drawn back). As a result I ate local breads and meats, dumplings, tomatoes, cucumber salads, chocolates and sweets. Meanwhile the 'phantom' pain on my right lower pain persisted and I was often sick with minor stomach ailments and problems with breathing. After living there for five years I returned to London and renewed acquaintance with all my old food favourites. That was when the real problems began.

After supper at friends' houses my stomach would

become so bloated that I looked pregnant, and I was regularly so tired that I had to immediately fall asleep after meals—I simply couldn't keep my eyes open. Those symptoms became a running joke with my friends and of course, at that time, I shared the joke. I didn't even think of my symptoms as evidence of something else, something far more serious. I just thought that's how I was and that was what my body did. But when the allergies and anaphylactic shock set in, I realised that I was up against something very big and serious and frightening.

After several months of Nystatin, Zinc and other supplements from Dr. Choy, including a mixture of specifically prepared and environmentally targeted allergy drops for hay fever, cats, dust etc., and a clear understanding of what foods to eat and what not to eat, I very slowly started to feel better, and to my amazement I felt much, much better. In fact, I felt better than I ever felt before in my life. I eliminated sugar from my diet completely, even citrus fruits, and I stopped eating bread. Instead I chose to focus on protein and vegetables, berries and selected carbohydrates. I consulted a dietician at the homeopathic hospital, who specialised in allergy cases like mine, and she introduced me to foods like quinoa and certain grains I had never heard of. She also gave me useful information about cooking certain foods and about allergy food-groups.

I was eating voraciously, slowly gaining confidence and feeling safe again. More than anything I was understanding how to keep my Candida under control, and as a result experiencing more wellness than I'd ever had before. I realised that my food cravings—especially those related to sugars—could almost be used as a barometer for the things I should avoid or keep an eye on. The bloating after meals stopped completely and even more remarkable, the lower right hand side stomach vanished along with my fatigue and other ailments. Today, I rarely get ill and am truly thankful to have met Dr. Choy. I literally cannot imagine where I would be had I not had his help. I've now been seeing him for about 20 years. For the first few years he needed to personally monitor my Candida levels and the supplements he was prescribing for me; now, though, I mostly visit his colleagues a few times a year to monitor environmental allergies such as hay fever and dust allergy.

Since seeing Dr. Choy I haven't taken a single antihistamine. I treat the environmental allergies with his drops, which help me through the few weeks a year I have symptoms. I am still very careful about what I eat, both for my wellbeing and to make sure I never again suffer anaphylaxis. Since I met Dr. Choy I've learnt how to cook, and now I love caring for what I put into my body and understanding how sugars affect me. From time to time I can eat a little ice cream or raw sugar, but I do so with moderation.

Thank you so much Dr. Choy, for the gift of wellbeing you've given me. And to readers who are sceptical or afraid of their current symptoms or allergy problems: I don't know if my story resonates with you, but if it does I strongly recommend you follow this book's advice.

Alice

10

FINAL WORDS

IN CONCLUSION

Candida overgrowth can account for a multitude of symptoms. Any symptom can have a relationship to the Candida problem whether it is strongly or weakly correlated but it must be remembered that other medical conditions can also give rise to those symptoms. The fact that one has a straightforward Candida problem may only be part of the story. Especially if the symptoms do not respond as expected, both doctor and patient must look for other reasons for the persistence of symptoms. It does not mean that just because you have a diagnosed Candida condition, you cannot also have a concomitant medical problem giving rise to your symptoms.

I remember a case that I saw twelve years ago and I want to share the story with you because it highlights the fact that we have to be alert to other factors.

SD whom I had seen and treated successfully for a Candida problem two years previously returned with a multitude of complaints saying that the Candida problem had returned. I listened to her carefully. Amongst her many symptoms, tiredness stood out prominently from the other complaints. The way she spoke about her tiredness and her body language suggested to me there might be more than just the Candida problem. I suggested a few standard tests and the first result to come back was a blood test which showed she had leukaemia. I am glad to say she was treated successfully for the leukaemia in her local general hospital. I saw her again five years later and her leukaemia had not recurred but she had a flare up of her Candida problem. I was not surprised that her Candida problem came on again because the chemotherapy used to treat the blood disease had affected her immune system and caused the flare up.

The next case is of somebody I saw more recently. He came with complaints of abdominal distention and he had heard from friends that Candida problems can cause tummy bloating, and that I see patients with such symptoms. When he walked into the room I could see that he was not well. On closer inspection, he looked jaundiced (yellowing of the skin), and after talking to him a bit more I realised that he certainly had problems with his liver. He was admitted to hospital where he was diagnosed as having cancer of the liver. I am glad to say he had surgery and treatment for the cancer and made a good recovery.

There is a condition called diverticulitis in which the diverticula (sacs or pouches usually in the large intestine) get inflamed and infected. This condition can present with abdominal symptoms like Candida. It occurs in older people and is usually treated with antibiotics. Occasionally patients present with fever and, rarely, it can cause an abdominal emergency when there is perforation of the intestine. Scans can confirm the presence of these diverticula. I am pleased to say that this is not so common. The reason for telling you all this is because other conditions can also be present alongside the Candida fermentation and we must be vigilant to it. Candida is not the only organism that ferments sugar. Bacteria also cause fermentation.

What to do

If you suspect your symptoms might be due to a Candida problem the first thing to do is to consult your doctor especially if you have multiple symptoms. You need tests to rule out other conditions which if present need to be treated in other ways. If tests do not come back positive and your doctor does not think your medical symptoms are due to anything ominous or if your symptoms are very mild, you can always try a diet excluding sugar first. A herbal antifungal would need to be taken as well to get the overgrowth under control. You should begin to feel better within ten days, though symptoms may still persist. If not, then exclude yeast and if there is really not much improvement then avoid wheat as well. Strict dieting for long periods is certainly not advisable. If you need to be on a strict diet to keep your symptoms under control then you need to see a doctor who has experience in treating Candida Overgrowth.

What to do if the symptoms persist

If, after a few months of treatment, the symptoms are still there then other tests will be required. I have had patients whose tummy symptoms persisted even though the Candida was treated and under control. I then recommend a comprehensive digestive stool analysis with parasitology. This is a stool test with faeces collected over three days which are sent to a laboratory in America that has the sophisticated instruments for a detailed analysis of the stools and the presence of parasites. The normal laboratories in the U.K cannot do such a detailed analysis although specialist research centres may have the necessary equipment. This test can show how the gut is functioning in terms of digestion and absorption, the levels of some beneficial bacteria, and if there is any degree of 'bad' bacteria causing symptoms and presence of parasites. Bacteria causing symptoms in the gut is well recognised in mainstream medicine. Small Intestine Bacteria Overgrowth (SIBO) needs to be treated by antibiotics though there are non-drug remedies used by non-medical practitioners. If parasites are also present, appropriate treatment must also be given. The results of such tests have so far helped me to treat those patients whose tummy symptoms did not subside simply with treatment of the Candida.

As you can see, Candida is a cause of many symptoms but it is not the only cause of a lot of symptoms. That said, when nothing seems to account for your complaints, then think of Candida. I have noticed that Candida Overgrowth is present in many unrelated medical conditions. I know that because I make it a point to ask about past medical history. Perhaps it is the stress associated with the medical condition that people have been diagnosed with, or the resultant treatment for the condition, I do not know. My guess is that, whatever that led to the development of the original condition can also cause the Candida problem. Even though the appropriate treatment for the original condition had been instituted and the original causative agent is long gone, they may be left with symptoms of the overgrowth. If that is sorted out, then patients can feel much better and maybe respond better to treatment for the concomitant medical condition.

11

FOOD STATE SUPPLEMENTS

NOT ALL NUTRITIONAL SUPPLEMENTS ARE THE SAME

You can get many nutritional supplements from any health food store, chemist, and most supermarkets even sell them. They are not all the same. Over the years I have used various types and brands of nutrients and found that they do not all produce the same end results. Some produce better results than other types or brands. The commonly available nutrients are all chemical isolates and as such they are not absorbed well with poor bioavailability (available to the body for use). Some compounds perform better than others. But they are all labelled 'natural' food supplements though they are nowhere near the nutrients we get from the foods we eat. Some doctors maintain that we do not need nutritional supplements if we eat properly. This is true to an extent but how many of us can truly say we eat properly and get in the right amount of nutrients at every meal? It is also true that the foods that we eat now do not contain the same amount of some nutrients as those foods did seventy years ago (this is according to data published by the government and is available at HMSO outlets). Also the pace of our lives is faster and more hectic than say one hundred years ago. For example, if we wanted to go to India in the past, it might have taken us up to a week to reach there by boat but now we can go on a plane and reach there in eight hours. Also with modern technology such as E-mail or video conference, we can get answers to our queries much faster and therefore have to act or perform at a much quicker pace than in the past. All these lead to more stress and therefore more nutrients are used up and faster to enable us to stay well and function properly. So when we are low in the nutrients in our body, then our response to the environment can be compromised.

I was introduced to food state supplements some twenty-eight years ago. The idea of a much more natural food supplement appealed to me a great deal but I must say that I initially used it with a degree of trepidation as yeast (saccharomyces cerevisiae) was involved in the manufacture of food state products. This fear was unfounded as I did not have any patients reporting adverse reaction from these supplements.

As I understand it, once the yeast cells have finished their role in the manufacturing process their cell walls are ruptured by the action of proteolytic enzymes added to them. This renders them unrecognisable as yeast molecules and therefore non allergenic. I have had a couple of patients who on seeing the word 'yeast' mentioned (even though there is no 'live' yeast present), despite assurances declined to take them. I have not any adverse reactions from these many yeast-sensitive patients. This I am glad to say is the exception (reluctance to take the recommended nutrients). Others were happy to take them and they have greatly benefited from them. In fact a few had remarked that when their supplements ran out they bought similar supplements from their local stores but did not get the same benefits from those as when they were having the food state supplements.

Our bodies are made to absorb nutrients from foods and not from chemicals. With non-food states the supplements are always in the form of chemical compounds. For example if you get Zinc it may be in the form of Zinc gluconate or Zinc oxide or citrate. Magnesium may be in the form of magnesium carbonate or magnesium sulphate. These are chemical compounds and such compounds do not occur naturally in our foods.

Pesticides which contain chemical compounds are different. They are added things and are not inherent in the foods we eat. There is for example Zinc and glucuronic acid in certain foods but not as a compound which is an entirely different substance. That is the way nutritional supplements have been prepared over the last fifty years at least. I suppose taking something with poorer absorption is better than taking nothing at all if you are deficient in those nutrients. If you take nothing extra you get zero extra of that nutrient. If you take something even though it is poorly absorbed, that which is absorbed into your body is definitely better than nothing extra. Hence people still derive some benefit from taking those non-food state supplements. What I am saying is that you can get even more benefit if you take a supplement that has been shown to be better absorbed and utilised by your body.

Nutrients from foods are what is best absorbed and utilised by the body, but if you are very low in certain nutrients it is not possible to eat enough of the foods that contain more of those nutrients. Some people do not eat oysters or shellfish which contain a high amount of Zinc naturally for all kinds of reasons. But even if you do eat them how many plates of oysters and shellfish can you eat without feeling fed up with the same foods everyday?

The next best thing in this context is food state supplements which I must stress are not food but are called food supplements.

Nutrients in foods are absorbed together with phospholipids, lipoproteins, amino acids, flavonoids, fatty acids and dietary fibres and carbohydrates and others. These co-factors aid the absorption and possibly make them more bioavailable to the body. The most significant difference in food state supplements is the presence of a vital carrier protein, a protein which helps to transport nutrients from food naturally across the cell membrane and deliver it to its intended site as nutrients in foods do. Chemical isolates do not have these co-factors and hence their absorption is less effective. It must be emphasised again that nutrients in foods have these factors which facilitate absorption and make them more available to the body for use.

I shall not lumber you with all the scientific jargon and details entailed in the manufacturing and preparation of the food state supplements. Instead I will explain the process to you in a non-scientific manner using a simple analogy (the way I understand it). Carrots grown in the soil will contain all the nutrients that carrots should. They can only get those nutrients from the soil but when the soil is exhausted of its nutrients it (the land) is left fallow, i.e. the land is not cultivated for 1-3 years to enable it to regain the nutrients naturally. That is how it was in the past. Nowadays with crop rotation, the next crop is waiting to be planted on the same patch of land. But the land is spent of nutrients. What to do? Fertilisers are added to enrich the soil but these are chemicals. The micro-organisms in the soil convert these

118

chemicals into something natural so that when the carrots take up those nutrients and when we eat the carrots we are no longer eating the original chemicals (fertilisers) that have been put in but nutrients from the carrots. In essence this is the similar principle to how food state supplements are prepared.

There is a lot of literature about food state supplements and their manufacture as well as many scientific comparative studies with other non food state supplements. I shall not go into details on that except to reiterate what the studies show and what the manufacturing company maintains.

1) better absorption

The food state materials in their phosphorylated protein form and the associated co-factors are in the same form as nutrients from foods which are naturally absorbed. Free state ionic forms (the chemicals isolates) need to be broken down and linked to a protein carrier before they can be absorbed. This requires cellular energy and so their absorption is usually unsatisfactory. In fact, compared with some chemicals isolates, the absorption rate of food state materials are several times better than their chemically derived counterparts.

2) increased availability (available to the body for use)

If you were to post a parcel to someone without putting an address it would hardly be surprising if that person did not receive it. It is the same with non-food state supplements. If they did not have the necessary co-factors (such as the phospholipids and lipoproteins etc) then the body could not absorb them efficiently. In the food state form with the associated and necessary co-factors the parcel would be delivered to the intended recipient. In several studies the bioavailability were much greater than the non-food state supplements.

3) decreased excretion in the urine,

4) increased retention in the cells

Both these above factors have enabled a lower dose to be used. Some patients think that a higher labelled dose such as Zinc Orotate 100mg is much more than Zinc in the food state form of 15 mg. This is not so. Firstly the elemental dose of Zinc in the 100mg of Orotate is no greater than 15mg. Secondly, because of its poorer absorption and lower retention in the body and the increased excretion in the urine, the effective dose is much less than the 15mg of Zinc in the food state form.

5) decreased toxicity

6) complete metabolism

7) does not block the absorption of other nutrients

Very often patients are told not to take one type of mineral with another as one can affect the absorption of the other. This is true. But remember the research leading to this conclusion was all done using chemical isolates. If you think about it, a meal contains all types of vitamins and minerals and you are never told that you cannot eat one type of food with another or the nutrients in those foods will interfere with each other's absorption. Nutrients from foods do not interfere with one another's absorption whereas nutrients from chemical isolates do. Similarly food state nutrients do not interfere with the absorption of other nutrients.

The above list is a synopsis of food state supplements and I must stress that the yeast used in the manufacturing process does not and has not affected any of my patients with a Candida problem. It is to be noted that Lactobaccillus Bulgaricus is now used in the manufacturing process instead of yeast in some nutrients and certainly in the production of Zinc and Magnesium and this has not reduced the efficacy of the products. This has certainly allayed anxiety in some patients who equate 'yeast' with their problem despite repeatedly being informed that the yeast used in the original manufacturing process is deactivated and harmless.

This chapter on food state supplements would not be complete without saying a few words about the man behind it, the discoverer Andrew Szalay.

In 1937 Albert Szent-Gyorgi,a professor at the University of Szeged in Hungary was awarded the Nobel prize for discovering and isolating Ascorbic Acid (Vitamin C). He also noted that the Ascorbic Acid that he isolated was not as active (not as bioavailable) as the Vitamin C contained in crushed paprika (red pepper) extract. This crucial and profound statement was overlooked and lost in the rush to discover and 'isolate' vitamins and minerals over the years.

Andrew Szalay also attended the University of Szeged, graduating in Pharmacy in 1946. He was consumed with the idea that if he could only produce vitamins and minerals in a more bioavailable form as his hero, Szent-Gyorgi had demonstrated, people could get superior nutrition without taking the large doses that scientists were recommending in trying to restore good health. He then set out to research and work on producing nutrients that would be well absorbed and acted in the body in the same way as nutrients from foods naturally would.

Finally, after a lifetime as a pharmacist and botanical scientist, he was able at the age of 58 to devote all his energy to developing a new form of nutrients. After many failures he succeeded in developing vitamins and minerals that have been shown to be different from 'isolated' supplements. The new nutrients were as close as possible to the natural food matrix and each nutrient was embedded in a matrix that had the greatest affinity with that specific nutrient. In 1977, by which time he was in New York, he established a company and began to market these nutrients. After two decades these products were being sold in over twent-five countries. These products were not only embraced by the nutrition companies but were also accepted and used by many pharmaceutical companies, food industries and cosmetic manufacturers. Twenty-eight years of ongoing scientific research, published scientific articles, testing in quality-control laboratories equipped with state of the art instrumentation and microbiological testing of every individual batch, all attest to the viability and superiority of these nutrients.

I hope that this has enabled you to see the difference between the various types of nutrients and why it is important to get the right type of food supplements in order to benefit from them maximally. The labels should carry the correct information.

12

DIETARY INFORMATION

SUGAR AND YEAST FREE

The information in this section is provided by Mrs. Joan Manning, nutritionist, whom I have known and worked with for a long time. I have just added some comments for patients, when I deem right to do so. As this is not a book about Candida diets the information given is just an overall view on what foods contains what. For those who need to do more dietary avoidance there is also information on what to avoid on a milk and wheat free diet.

Sugar

The obvious sugar and things containing sugar or made with them are obviously not allowed.

All fruits and vegetable contain to a variable extent fructose (fruit sugar). Those with amounts:

greater than 20 percent of sugar – HIGH

They include all the dried fruits like apricots, currants, dates, figs, peaches, prunes, raisins and sultanas. Though honey is not a fruit, it contains a high amount of fructose and may contain added sugar.

10-20 percent – MEDIUM

Grapes, melons, bananas,apples, bilberry, cherry, lychee, nectarine, pear, pineappleand pomegranate.

5 -10 percent – LOW

This generally include various berries, lemon and lime.

Less than 5 percent – VERY LOW

This includes other common fruits and vegetables eaten in the western hemisphere. Some vegetables commonly give rise to bloating such as garlic, onion, beans and those from the cabbage family, but patients will be alright with them when the Candida is sorted out.

Yeast-containing foods

Not necessary in majority of patients that I have seen with the Candida problem. If they also have yeast sensitivity then it is important for them to be aware of the foods in this list:

Grains: Bread, rolls, buns, doughnuts, Danish pastry. Some pancakes are made with yeast (blinis). Much patisserie has yeast as an ingredient. Many breakfast cereals have malt (yeast).

Meat: All breaded products eg. fish fingers,chicken Kiev

Fish: Many raised pies. Ready-cooked casseroles. Burgers,

Fowl: Sausages, soups and stock cubes, gravy and processed products.

Vegetables: Mushrooms. Any fermented vegetable like sauerkraut.

Pickles.

Fruits: Dried fruits. Grapes and all over-ripe fruits.

Citrus fruit juice (unless freshly squeezed).

Dairy: Cheese and all fermented milk products such as soured cream and buttermilk.

Nuts: 'Wet'nuts and undried walnuts. Peanuts and pistachios.

Beverages: All alcoholic drinks (yeast is used to ferment sugar into alcohol). Commercially prepared citrus fruit juices. Tea and herb tea. Malted milk drink

Yeast drinks.

Condiments:

Citric acid (maybe derived from fermentation with additives such as Aspergillus Niger).

Soy sauce, vinegar and product containing vinegar such salad dressings, pickles, ketchups, sweet and sour sauces, Marmite, Bovril, other yeast extract drinks,barbecue sauces and stock cubes and monosodium glutamate.

Mint sauce

Hot spices and curries

Soya: there are now many soy products in products being used as replacements for dairy foods.

Please remember that substitute 'cheeses' and 'yoghurts' together with tofu and other fermented soya products should be avoided.

The following foods are associated with Moulds, or quickly become mouldy. Some may already have been listed with the 'yeasty' foods:

Vegetables: all root vegetables(as moulds are found in the soil). These vegetables should be peeled and cleaned carefully. If you wish to eat jacket potatoes, you should thoroughly scrub the potato, boil for two or three minutes, then proceed to bake it. Mushroom and truffles (the vegetable kind) should be avoided.

Dairy: cheese, all fermented milk & soya milk products, soured milk.

Nuts: peanuts,pistachio and all 'wet'nuts.

Nuts can be dried in the oven for about twenty minutes and then kept in an airtight container.

Antibiotics: many are derived from moulds though there are also many synthetic forms of antibiotics.

N.B. All over-ripen fruits and vegetables will have a tendency to grow moulds.

All refrigerated dishes – meat, fish, salads, vegetables etc will eventually attract moulds.

It is therefore wise to eat food as fresh as possible.

What you are allowed to eat:
FRESH. Meats, fish,fowl and eggs.
GRAINS.

i) Wheat, shredded wheat, pasta, yeast-free bread (soda bread), scones, pastry, crackers, matzos and flour products without added yeast.

ii) Rye – crisp bread such as Ryvita and Ryking.

iii) Oats – porridge,oatcakes and oatmeal.

iv) Maize – cornflour,cornmeal, sweetcorn and other corn products without yeast.

v) Rice – all sorts of rice,rice cakes,rice pasta, rice cereals and flour.

vi) Buckwheat/quinoa/sago/tapioca
Dairy. Milk,'live'yoghurt and buttermilk.

Fruits & Vegetables: they must be fresh. Grapes are not allowed.

Nuts:all except peanuts and pistachios.

Fats & Oils: vegetable oils, margarines and spreads.

Seeds: sesame,sunflower etc.

Some suggested yeast and sugar free food items you may like to eat:
BREAKFAST. You may choose any from:
Yeast free bread,toasted or untoasted,with butter or spread.

126

Cereal – any sugar free especially porridge topped with a few berries.

Rice cakes, oatcakes and corn cakes.

Eggs – boiled,scrambled or omelette.

Pate (read label if not home-made).

Cold sliced meats (not preserved meats like salami).

Avocado stuffed with prawns or sliced with tomato and cold chicken breast.

Kedgree (if bought read label)

Smoothie – made from yoghurt and topped with bran.

Drinks: water(with a slice of lemon), coffee or tea but no sugar, permitted juices – diluted.

LUNCH

It is always awkward if you can't 'grab a sandwich' if you are not at home or at work. Most of our light lunches or snacks seem to be sandwiches,rolls or wraps. However, here are some ideas:

i) soup with a yeast free roll,bread or crackers.

ii) any plain meat or fish. If you want fish and chips ask for it to be grilled or pan fried without batter.

iii) jacket potato with tuna, butter or allowed fillings.

iv) salad – choice of vegetables and cold meat, fish or eggs. Dress with olive oil,sesame or walnut.

v) stir fry – use sesame oil and a little chicken stock (home-made) instead of soy sauce.

vi) omelette with choice of filling (not cheese)

vii) choice of mezze: stuffed vine leaves, humus, tzatziki, yeast-free pitta bread etc.

viii) of course, you can have sandwich made from yeast-free bread or roll.

You can have sugar-free yoghurt or a piece of fruit for dessert.

DINNER

Starter from: soup (home made preferably as you know what is in it). Otherwise a clear chicken soup or beef broth is probably safest. Or a good home made vegetable soup.

Grapefruit

Salad leaves with avocado,smoked salmon,tomato cucumber, dressed with flavoured oil and garnished with choice of herbs.

Pate (check label) and eat with crackers

Tempura vegetables,prawns with mus-sized strips or wedges (carrots, celery, cucumber, baby sweetcorn, broccoli) with an assortment of dips (aubergine, humus, egg & watercress, tomato relish, guacamole etc)

Barbecue chicken wings

Main dish from:

any roasted, grilled, braised or stewed meat or chicken

any fish – pan-fried,steamed,or baked in oven.

any stir fry using flavoured oils instead of soy sauce and without mushroom.

any pasta or spaghetti without cheese.

any rice dish or risotto without cheese.

any vegetable dish without mushroom.

any egg dish without cheese or mushroom.

Dessert from:

any permitted fresh fruit

profiteroes filled with unsweetened cream, dusted with cocoa powder.

crumble made with fruits with no added sugar (topping include cinnamon or other spices in the crumble mix and sprinkled with grated or flaked almond)

pancakes made without sugar and stuffed with

strawberries or raspberries and cream.

bake sugar-free pastry case 'blind'. Fill with berries or sliced poached fruit. Brush with sugar free jelly made a little thicker than usual. Leave to set. Serve with a little pureed fruit.

mix a thick sugar-free yoghurt with a little fruit of choice (shredded pineapple, berries, poached plums, apricots, peaches or cherries, cut into small pieces) and chill in the freezer for about half an hour. Serve. If you leave in the freezer too long it will set solid.

sugar-free rice pudding – served hot or cold with grated nutmeg.

NOTES:
You may drink sugar-free mixers if you feel too limited by drinking water. If they are served with a couple of ice cubes and a slice of orange or lemon, they will look like a drink that can be enjoyed.

If you really have to use a sweetener – most makers will provide recipes for cooking or baking with them.

Instead of soy sauce use either sesame or walnut oil.

They are both highly flavoured. Don't buy too much in one go as they should be used as fresh as possible for the best taste.

If you want to make your own fishcake or meatballs,use mashed potato as a binder instead of bread.

You will note that as long as you eat sugar-free foods and avoid bread, cheese, mushroom and strong spices there are many dishes that can be prepared and eaten.

HISTORICAL PERSPECTIVE II

SOCIETIES IN MANY COUNTRIES DEALING WITH ENVIRONMENTAL MEDICINE

For those readers interested in the progression and later widespread use of the approach used in dealing with patients with various unexplained symptoms by doctors doing clinical ecology—subsequently called environmental medicine physicians—I have outlined the development here.

The story of Herbert Rinkel and the development of the intradermal technique is relevant to know, so that the progression and views of this approach to a very common problem can be understood.

A group of like-minded doctors in USA came together in the early 1970s to practice this clinical ecology approach. It was found that many patients with hitherto bizarre symptoms that used to baffled doctors could be understood using this approach. The Miller technique of testing and treatment was found to be effective in the management of these patients.

With increasing success and more doctors attracted to this approach the American Academy of Environmental Medicine was formed some 25 years ago replacing the confusing term of clinical ecology. A list of doctors in different states in the USA who practice this approach is available from the Academy.

Around the mid 1970s this concept came to the UK and a group of doctors who subscribe to this approach formed the clinical ecology group. The doctors of this group have increased rapidly and the name of this society has now changed to BSAENM (British Society for Allergy, Environmental and Nutritional Medicine).

There are also doctors in Europe who practise this approach and this has also spread to Australia.

USEFUL ADDRESSES

Vitamins & Minerals levels measurement.
Biolab Medical Unit
The Stone House
9 Weymouth Street
London W1N 3FF
Tel: 0207 636 5959

Comprehensive digestive stools analysis:
Genova Diagnostics
Parkgate House
356 West Barnes Lane
New Malden
Surrey KT3 6NB
Tel: 0208 336 7750

Food-state nutritional supplements:
Oriental & Western Ltd (OWL)
Unit 26 Langston Priory Workshops
Station Road
Kingham Oxon
OX7 6UP
Tel: 01608 659925

Candida treatment:
Nightingale Clinic
Lister House
11-12 Wimpole Street
London W1G 9ST
Tel: 0207 436 2135